The 7 Secrets of Sound Healing

Books

Healing Sounds
Shifting Frequencies
The Lost Chord
Tantra of Sound (with Andi Goldman)

Music CDs

Trance Tara
Sacred Gateways
Dolphins Dreams
Chakra Chants (vol. 1 and 2)
The Divine Name* (with Gregg Braden)
Holy Harmony
Celestial Yoga
Reiki Chants
The Angel and the Goddess
The Lost Chord
De-Stress
Waves of Light
Celestial Reiki (vol. 1 and 2; with Laraaji and Sarah Benson)
Frequencies
ChakraDance
Medicine Buddha
Ultimate Om
Tantra of Sound Harmonizer (with Andi Goldman)

Instructional CDs

Healing Sounds Instructional
Vocal Toning the Chakras

DVD

Healing Sounds

*Available from Hay House

Please visit Hay House USA: **www.hayhouse.com**®
Hay House Australia: **www.hayhouse.com.au**
Hay House UK: **www.hayhouse.co.uk**
Hay House South Africa: **www.hayhouse.co.za**
Hay House India: **www.hayhouse.co.in**

The 7 Secrets of Sound Healing

JONATHAN GOLDMAN

HAY HOUSE, INC.
Carlsbad, California • New York City
London • Sydney • Johannesburg
Vancouver • Hong Kong • New Delhi

Hay House, Inc.: www.hayhouse.com • Hay House Australia Pty. Ltd.: www.hayhouse.com. au • Hay House UK, Ltd.: www.hayhouse.co.uk • Hay House SA (Pty), Ltd.: • www.hayhouse. co.za • Raincoast: www.raincoast.com • Hay House Publishers India: www.hayhouse.co.in

Editorial supervision: Jill Kramer • *Design:* Charles McStravick

Photographs of water crystals from Dr. Masaru Emoto reprinted with permission of I.H.M. General Institute: **www.hado.net**.
CymaGlyphs® created by Erik Larson, in collaboration with John Stuart Reid, inventor of the CymaScope™.

Library of Congress Control Number: 2006932599

Tradepaper ISBN: 978-1-4019-3792-8

14 13 12 11   7 6 5 4
1st edition, March 2008
4th edition, December 2011

Printed in the United States of America

To Sarah Benson,
the "Divine Mother of Sound Healing,"
who taught me that
the true sound of healing
is Love.

· · ·

Contents

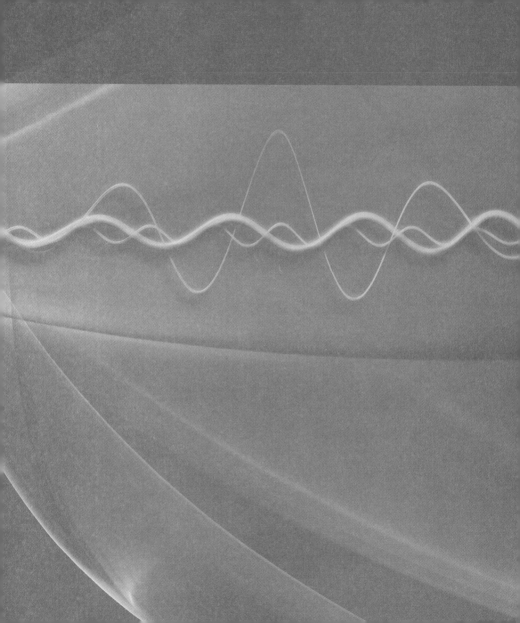

Preface

I used to be a walking encyclopedia of sound healing. Through the years, though, I've forgotten more than I can remember. I suppose that this is because the more experiences I personally had with sound, the less meaningful all the factual information that I'd obtained then seemed. That still remains true for me today—the real teaching is *the sound.*

The 7 Secrets of Sound Healing is the result of more than 25 years of study, research, teaching, and experience in the field of sound healing. I wrote it in order to honor *the sound* and the extraordinary transformation that it has brought me . . . and in order to assist you, the reader, in understanding the true healing power of sound.

The psychic Edgar Cayce predicted that the medicine of the future would be sound. And, indeed, we are moving into that future. As we do so, more and more information—and misinformation—about sound and its healing ability is beginning to manifest. Thus, I've written *The 7 Secrets of Sound Healing* to provide some understanding of the myriad different forms that this modality has taken.

I have a Master of Arts degree in the Independent Study of the Uses of Sound and Music for Healing from Lesley University in Cambridge, Massachusetts, the result of my having founded the Sound Healers Association in 1982—an organization dedicated to research and awareness of this subject. Every month different people, such as doctors, scientists, musicians, and spiritual masters, would come and give freely of their time, lecturing to a group of interested individuals I'd assembled. These presenters were the true pioneers in the field of sound healing. While many of their names may be forgotten today, they gave me the foundation for the information, techniques, exercises, and knowledge that I'm presenting to you.

As a result of their teaching, I ultimately pursued the master's-degree program at Lesley University, which led me to write my first book and gave me the confidence to present my first lecture. During this studying, writing, and then teaching,

I also continued to play and create music for healing, meditation, and relaxation.

Why sound healing? My story begins one night in 1980 in a seaside bar in the town of Marshfield, Massachusetts, where I was in a rock 'n' roll band. I'd been performing in various groups since I'd first taught myself to play guitar after watching the Beatles on *The Ed Sullivan Show.* That night in 1980, however, something happened: While performing, I became aware that—besides the alcohol and other intoxicants that were being imbibed by the patrons of the club—the music that my band and I were creating was contributing to an ambience of negativity. Then I had the thought: *What if music could be used to make people feel better?* The concept of using sound to heal didn't enter my psyche until a few weeks later. But that thought—that question about sound, and more specifically, music, being used to make people feel good—completely changed my life.

Soon after, I began to research information on all aspects of sound as a healing and transformative modality. This was back in the early 1980s, when the Internet didn't yet exist and specialized information (and misinformation) wasn't so easy to come by. But if there was an esoteric bookstore in any town I passed through, I would find it.

Through the founding of the Sound Healers Association, I was able to gain access to even more arcane information about sound. I'm a pretty good autodidact . . . I like to teach myself—and I certainly did of lot of that, as well as taking lessons in everything from the physics of sound to the creation of vocal harmonics. And, as I said, those extraordinary people who came to present at the meetings I held carried with them a wealth of knowledge that they were only too eager to share. In my "birth" and upbringing in this field of sound, I was weaned and nurtured by some of the best teachers on the planet, including Dr. Randall McClellan, Kay Gardner, Don Campbell, Dr. Peter Guy Manners, Sarah Benson, Steven Halpern, Dr. John Beaulieu, and others too numerous to cite.

I remember giving my first lecture on sound healing in the mid-'80s, sharing with the audience my understanding of what it would take to truly comprehend the realm of sound. My notes read:

> *In order to fully research, investigate, understand, and use the power of sound and music as therapeutic tools, one would need to be:*

> 1. *Physician—understanding the mechanism of the body*

> 2. *Physicist—understanding the mechanism of energy*

> 3. *Psychologist—understanding the process of behavior*

4. *Psychoacoustician—understanding the effects of sound on the brain*

5. *Audiologist—understanding the mechanism of the ear and hearing*

6. *Acupuncturist—understanding Oriental medicine*

7. *Ethnomusicologist—understanding the ethnic history and origins of music*

8. *Mathematician—understanding the mathematics of music*

9. *Philosopher—understanding the concepts behind music's creation and use*

10. *Linguist—understanding the various aspects of language*

11. *Neurologist—understanding the mechanisms of the nervous system and brain*

12. *Electrical engineer—understanding the building of instrumentation*

13. *Magician—understanding the use of chants and magical formulas*

14. *An expert trained in all the esoteric and spiritual subjects*

15. *A healer trained in all traditions, including chakras, bioenergy, and etheric fields*

16. *A shaman, able to induce and travel to different states of consciousness*

17. *A musician trained on many instruments to read and improvise*

18. *A vocalist, able to create all techniques of singing, chanting, and toning.*

In hindsight, it's apparent to me that there are many more categories that could be included in the preceding list, but it was obvious to me and everyone else in the audience that night that it was truly impossible for any individual to be sufficiently versed in all these different modalities of learning. One could engage in sound healing and experience great benefits, but not be a master in *all* of the various categories. Thus, the reality of being a full-fledged "sound healer" was not to be had—at least not in this lifetime. To be proficient in even one of the categories I mentioned would take most of a person's waking hours. Therefore, no single human could possibly do this. The world of sound healing was like an extraordinary pie in which we all could have a piece (or even two) if we were diligent—but no one could know everything. It was that simple.

Fast-forward 20 years, and the world of sound healing is reaching mainstream consciousness. There are articles in *The New York Times,* segments on national TV shows, and mass-marketed speakers all imparting knowledge about the power of sound to heal and transform. It's important for audiences exposed to this information to be able to discern what's valid about sound from what isn't.

Thus, the need for this book—short, simple, and (hopefully) full of much truth. While, from my perspective, it may still be impossible for any one person to be fully versed in the multifaceted aspects of sound healing, there's no reason why everybody can't have some awareness and understanding of it. In addition, *anyone* can receive extraordinary benefits from delving into this form of healing . . . and learning to use sound for stress and pain reduction, relaxation, sleep enhancement, and much more, as will be explored later in these pages. So, I present to you *The 7 Secrets of Sound Healing.*

The book is divided into seven easy-to-understand chapters that will help you recognize some of the basic principles of sound healing. It will also allow you to apply practical exercises in order to experience this modality for yourself. My ultimate aim in this endeavor is for the 7 Secrets revealed herein to open you up to the world of sound healing so that you can use the information, exercises, knowledge, and techniques to lead a healthier, happier life. That's my intention, and I trust it will manifest for all who are reading this book.

Thank you for accompanying me on this most marvelous journey into the realms of healing and transformation through sound. Hop on board. We're about to ride the wave of sound!

· · ● ● ● · ·

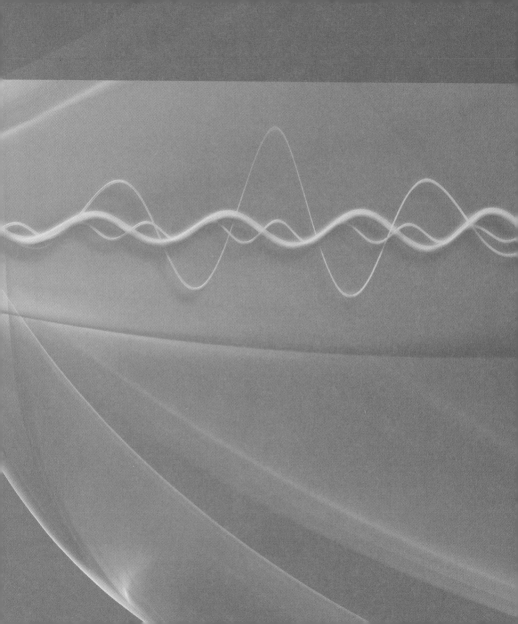

Introduction

*T*he *7 Secrets of Sound Healing* provides an important framework of basic knowledge to anyone interested in the field of sound healing. The information contained in these pages will allow you to investigate and benefit from the various modalities that are currently available. You'll receive an understanding of just what may be experienced in this ever-expanding domain. This work presents techniques and exercises that you can practice at home using the power of sound for wellness and self-transformation. By applying these exercises, as well as listening to the accompanying

CD, you'll be able to immediately experience sound healing for yourself.

My intention in writing this book is to provide a means by which readers can begin to understand the various aspects and uses of sound as a healing modality. The reason for this is quite simple: The world of sound healing is growing. It's not uncommon to pick up a magazine and find an article about some application of sound either to mend the physical body or transform the psyche. Such a discussion of sound might be heard on a radio show or via other forms of media. The question is: How can this be? How can sound be used to heal and transform? *The 7 Secrets of Sound Healing* presents you with answers to these questions in seven clear and coherent chapters, each one revealing a specific secret of sound healing.

Sound is routinely used in different areas of medicine and holistic healing and counseling. It's common practice for a doctor to harness it in the form of ultrasound in order to create images of a fetus for parents to view. Ultrasound is also available as a treatment for kidney stones as well as for the acceleration of healing of bone fractures. It's currently being tested experimentally for use with cancer patients. There are scientists who have examined our genetic code, found it analogous to music, and are researching ways in which sound may be able to effect healing through our

DNA. Sound is now commonly being used in traditional allopathic as well as complementary medicine to help ease pain and relieve stress.

Are you experiencing fatigue, feeling anxious, or having trouble sleeping? Your health practitioner might suggest a particularly relaxing CD to help alleviate your problem. Is your child experiencing difficulties in school? A learning-disability expert might suggest a highly advanced system of stimulating sounds, which have proven helpful in assisting those with problems in the classroom. Are you going to a physical therapist or a chiropractor for a physical difficulty? You might find that your treatment includes a device that projects frequencies into your body to heal your muscles or tendons or even to align your vertebrae.

If you visit a massage therapist, you'll probably find that your session is accompanied by some very calming music playing in the background. Go to a holistic psychotherapist, and he or she may use music to help induce deep relaxation or use some sort of sound to balance the hemispheres of your brain and lower your brain-wave activity.

Medical visionaries such as Deepak Chopra, M.D., have proclaimed, "The universe is sound!" They tell us that our bodies are orchestras that can be tuned and made healthy with music, mantras, and many other sonic modalities. Andrew Weil, M.D., whose many books and recordings include *Self-Healing with Sound & Music,* informs us that sound therapy has been found effective in treating a surprising range of health challenges, including heart disease, arthritis, stress, emphysema, and more. In conjunction with his traditional medical practice, Mitchell Gaynor, M.D., the author of *Sounds of Healing,* uses the tones of quartz-crystal bowls and Tibetan metal bowls with his patients to calm and relax them.

With so much interest in this modality, it's necessary to become aware of the *how?* and *why?* of sound healing and to discriminate between what's effective and what isn't. It's important to have a basic understanding of the way sound healing works—which is what this book allows for.

As I mentioned, *The 7 Secrets of Sound Healing* is divided into seven chapters, each of which explores a specific secret of sound healing that I've discovered. The first four provide a basic understanding of how sound can be used to heal and transform. The last three offer practical ways that you can apply this knowledge to enhance your daily life.

— **Secret 1** is: "Everything Is Vibration." Here you'll discover the first principle on which both modern physicists and ancient mystics can agree—that everything is in a state of vibration. Your body is like an orchestra that can be tuned with sound. You'll find out about *frequency,* discover the phenomena of *resonance* and *entrainment,* and come to a basic understanding of how sound can be used to heal and transform.

— **Secrets 2** is: "Intent Is Powerful." The universe is in a state of vibration, and how these vibrations interact with you depends not only upon their actual frequency, but also the *intent* or the energy behind the frequency that's sounded. With this secret you'll learn the importance of your thoughts, feelings, and beliefs and how they may be used to amplify the healing power of sound.

— **Secret 3** is: "We Are All Unique Vibratory Beings." In this chapter, your individuality is honored as well as your own personal reaction to sound as you discover factors that may influence its effects. You'll understand how these effects may be very different for each of us. With this secret you'll realize that there is no single sound that's a cure-all for everything and everyone.

— **Secret 4** is: "Silence Is Golden." Here you'll explore another principle—the importance of silence in the process of sound healing. You'll also examine the concept of sound amplitude through the discovery that sound is a subtle energy. This chapter will impart to you the essential understanding that just because something is louder doesn't mean that it's more effective in creating healing.

— **Secret 5** is: "Our Voice Is the Most Healing Instrument." In this chapter, you'll discover a very important secret—that we each have the most extraordinary sound-healing instrument: our voice. With this chapter, you'll begin to apply in practice the principles you've explored. You'll learn to use your voice in a technique called *toning* to resonate with your chakras, bringing yourself balance and healing.

— **Secret 6** is: "There Are Many Notes in a Scale." Just as there are many different sounds that can be created from a musical instrument, so there are numerous diverse approaches to using sound as a healing system. This secret focuses on a dozen of the major applications of sound to heal and transform. You'll learn about the different modalities and what you might hope to experience through each of them.

— **Secret 7** is: "Sound Can Change the World." With this secret you'll discover that sound, coupled with consciousness, may be used to help co-create reality. Here you'll realize sound's importance not only as an extraordinary tool for healing yourself, but also for healing the planet. You'll learn how to apply this knowledge to assist in creating peace and harmony on a global level.

I invite you to use *The 7 Secrets of Sound Healing* as a practical guide to sound healing, opening yourself up to the many wonders that it can manifest. Allow this book to bring sound's extraordinary power to you. You'll find that it can heal and transform, enhancing your well-being, heightening your consciousness, and bringing balance and harmony into your daily life.

· · ● ● ● · ·

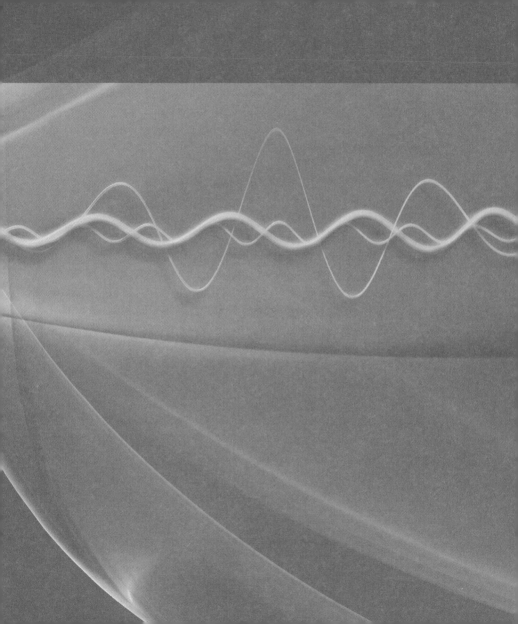

Everything
Is
Vibration

The first secret of sound healing has been known by mystics, healers, and spiritual teachers since ancient times. It's a secret that provides the basis for all the others in this book, and is now being echoed in the words of visionary doctors and quantum physicists, who—like the ancient mystics—declare that the world is sound. The first secret is this: *Everything is in a state of vibration.*

If you examine the basic tenets of the planet's different religions and spiritual paths, each has an understanding that the world was created through sound. Some examples include:

- In the book of Genesis, from the Old Testament, one of the first statements is: "And God said, 'Let there be light.'"

- In the Gospel according to John, from the New Testament, it is written: "In the beginning was the Word, and the Word was with God, and the Word was God."

- From the Vedas of the Hindu tradition comes the writing: "In the beginning was Brahman with whom was the Word. And the Word is Brahman."

- The ancient Egyptians believed that the god Thoth created the world by his voice alone.

- The Hopi Indians tell the story of Spider Woman, who sang the Song of Creation over the inanimate forms on Earth, bringing them to life.

- In the Australian Aboriginal tradition, the sound of the didgeridoo was responsible for creating the world.

- Many African legends from different tribes tell of the origin of the world through sound.

- According to the sacred Mayan text the *Popol Vuh,* the first humans were given life solely through the power of the word.

- In Polynesia and the Far East, the gods and goddesses struck gongs or blew conch shells in order to create the world.

In addition to the various sacred texts of this planet that describe sound as the major force of manifestation, the ancient mystery schools that existed thousands of years ago in Rome, Athens, Egypt, India, China, and Tibet had vast knowledge of the power of sound to heal. The various writings that have survived from those times indicate that in such traditions the use of sound as a therapeutic tool was a highly developed spiritual science, based upon an understanding that vibration was the fundamental creative force of the universe.

In India, there's a saying: "Nada Brahman"—the world is sound! The words of the ancients are now echoing those of our top scientists, such as quantum physicist Michio Kaku, who has declared, "Everything is music." Modern physics, in fact, tells us that this dimension and others are actually composed of tiny strings that vibrate at different rates.

FREQUENCY

Let's begin our discussion with some very simple and basic concepts about sound. First, it's currently understood as being a wave. Usually, this wave manifests as moving air, which takes the vibrations of an object and causes them to travel. This wave of sound strikes our eardrums and goes through the most extraordinary bioacoustic process in which it's first transformed into chemical form and then into electrical impulses as it travels through our brain.

Sound waves are measured in cycles per second. Scientifically, these cyclical wave measurements are called *hertz* and are abbreviated as *Hz*. The measurement of a sound is called its *frequency*. One cycle per second is written as 1 Hz. Extremely slow waves create very deep, bass sounds; extremely fast ones create very high, treble sounds. The lowest note on a piano is around 24 waves per second (24 Hz), and the highest is just over 4,000 (4,186 Hz, to be exact).

We have the ability to hear from around 16 Hz to around 16,000 Hz. These numbers, of course, aren't constant, particularly the upper measurements of our ability to hear. Young children are said to be able to hear upwards of 20,000 Hz, but as we grow older and our exposure to loud sounds increases, our range *de*creases. Sounds below our threshold of hearing are often called *infrasound,* while those above our audible range are referred to as *ultrasound.*

Years ago, I went with my son and his second-grade class to the Multisensory Sound Lab at the University of Colorado's Fiske Planetarium. This amazing room was conceived of by Norman Lederman, a colleague of mine, who wanted to create a place where hearing-impaired children could experience sound. It's really a fun place to visit. There are sound speakers under the floor, and if you talk into the microphone that connects to them, the floor vibrates. There's also a color organ that flashes different shades when various notes are played on it. Another interesting experiment involves a frequency generator (a scientific device that creates specific sounds), which is used to demonstrate our range of hearing.

I remember the instructor at the Multisensory Sound Lab saying, "Now, this is a frequency of 12,000 Hz. How many of you can hear it?" And everybody in the room, both children and parents, raised their hands.

The instructor continued: "13,000 Hz?" All of us kept our hands up.

"14,000 Hz?" A few of the more elderly in the room dropped their hands.

"15,000 Hz?" More adult hands were lowered.

"16,000 Hz?" Still more hands dropped. I was one of the few adults whose hand still waved with all the children.

Now, I pride myself on having extraordinarily sensitive ears, despite too many youthful years of playing electric guitar and listening to loud music. I like to believe that I can hear a pin drop in the next room. And maybe I can—but not if that pin is dropping at a frequency of 17,000 Hz, which was the next one that was demonstrated.

"17,000 Hz?" the instructor asked.

I heard nothing. I looked at my son. "You can hear that?" I asked. He nodded his head and smiled. From then on, until the instructor stopped demonstrating at 20,000 Hz, all the younger children continued with their hands up in the air. I still heard nothing. Neither could anyone else in the room who had reached beyond their teenage years. For me, it was a startling lesson regarding something that I'm going to share with you now.

Just because we can't hear something doesn't mean that there isn't a sound. It's that simple! And for the remainder of this book, and hopefully for the rest of your life, I'm going to ask you to do something: perceive sound as being much greater than the small bandwidth of frequencies that fall within your audible range. Our cetacean friends in the ocean, the dolphins, can receive and project frequencies upwards of 180,000 Hz. That's nearly ten times our highest level of hearing. When these sea creatures communicate, they exchange many levels of information at extraordinarily high rates of speed. To us, there's nothing happening; but to these dolphins, they may be sharing tuna haute cuisine with each other—or perhaps the best route through the Bering Strait!

To repeat: Just because we can't hear something doesn't mean there isn't anything there.

I've had students who claimed all sorts of sensitivity to sound, and I have no reason to doubt them. I've encountered those who could hear the sound of an electric current running through a house or that of a seemingly silent lamp as it burned bright. One student could hear different frequencies coming from various quartz crystals, while another could pick up on actual tones emitted by the body. I heard nothing, but that doesn't mean that these sounds weren't there.

As the ancient mystics declared, "Everything is sound!" From the electrons moving around the nucleus of an atom to the planets in distant galaxies revolving around stars, everything is in state of vibration—and therefore, conceptually at least, everything is creating a sound. Whether or not we can hear these sounds is another story.

RESONANCE

Resonance is the natural vibration of an object—the specific frequency at which it vibrates. Every object has a resonant frequency, whether or not we can hear it audibly. This book has a resonant frequency, as do the individual pages. The chair you might be sitting on has one; so does the glass from which you may be drinking.

There are two separate categories of resonance. The first is called "free resonance"—when an object will begin to vibrate only when it comes in contact with a frequency that exactly matches its own. This is true, for example, with tuning forks. If you have a fork of a certain frequency (let's say, 100 Hz), then strike another with this same frequency and bring it near the original one, the first will begin to vibrate and sound along with the second, struck one. In fact, you can put ten tuning forks of the same resonant frequency (100 Hz) near each other, strike just one of them, bring it near the others . . . and all ten of the unstruck tuning forks will sound. However, if you change the frequency of that first tuning fork by even 1 Hz—so that it now has a vibration of 101 Hz—there will be no resonance with any of those of 100 Hz. When you bring this first tuning fork near them, the others will no longer sound.

The second category of resonance is called "forced resonance." This occurs when one vibrating source produces vibrations in another object even though those two objects may not share the exact same frequency. Thus, the vibrations of one can entrain or change those of the other. Vibrating sources that are subject to the influence of "forced resonance" will resonate with many different frequencies.

As Dr. Randall McClellan has noted in *The Healing Forces of Music,* water is an example of a substance that responds to forced resonance, as are all the different materials from which we construct our musical instruments. We can, for example, hit many different notes on a violin, piano, or guitar and hear them all. Of great significance in the world of sound healing is the fact that the human body is a complex vibratory system that also resonates in this manner, responding to all sorts of different frequencies.

There are many frequencies that affect us and to which we can resonate. The various parts of our bodies—our organs, bones, tissues, and different bodily systems—all have their own specific resonant frequencies. Together, these frequencies create a composite harmonic: our own personal resonance or vibratory rate. We're like an extraordinary orchestra that's playing and creating the "Suite of the Self." When we're in a state of wellness and are performing this wonderful "Suite of the Self," we call this condition of balance and harmony *sound health.* However, what happens if the second-violin player loses his or her sheet music and begins to hit the wrong notes—the wrong harmony and melody? Soon not only is this musician playing out of tune, but he or she is also playing out of time and the whole string section sounds off, affecting the entire orchestra.

When a portion of the body is vibrating out of ease and out of harmony, we call this condition "dis-ease." I come from a family of physicians (my father, grandfather, and brother are all medical doctors), and I have the greatest respect for traditional allopathic medicine. But continuing with the metaphor of the body being like an orchestra, allopathic medicine would deal with the string player who'd lost his or her sheet music by either giving this poor individual enough drugs to pass out and no longer play; or else, analogous to surgery, cutting his or her head off with a sword. These steps obviously remove the out-of-tune musician, and those wrong notes that were so poorly affecting the orchestra are no longer present . . . but neither is the second-violin player! What if it were instead possible to somehow restore the sheet music to this person? What if we could somehow project the correct resonant frequency to whatever part of the body was vibrating out of ease and out of harmony?

This is the very basis of sound healing, and it's fundamental to our understanding of the use of sound to heal and transform. It's simple and it makes much sense—and it's all based on the concept that everything is in a state of vibration, including the body. Almost every modality of sound healing utilizes the approach of enhancing the correct resonant frequency of a part of the physical, emotional, mental, or spiritual body. When applied to the physical self, these resonant frequencies have the ability to charge the energy of failing cells, bringing them back to a state of health. In later chapters, I'll discuss the application of different modalities of sound healing, but regardless of whether the technique involves an electronic device, an acoustic instrument, or the human voice, most often it uses this concept of resonant-frequency healing, in which the natural, healthy vibrations are restored.

Through rejuvenating and restoring the body's own resonant frequencies, any imbalance ceases and healing occurs. This principle of resonant frequency is employed in the most common methods of sound healing. There is, however, one additional approach to sound, which is currently being applied in modern medicine—using frequencies to eradicate unwanted rogue cells and dissolve substances, such as crystallized minerals in the kidneys. This technique is also applied in more innovative sound healing to rid the body of unwanted bacteria, viruses, and fungi.

In the Old Testament story of Joshua and the walls of Jericho, after several days of encircling the city while beating drums and blowing horns, Joshua's men "shouted a great shout" and the walls collapsed. Some of you may recall a television commercial in which Ella Fitzgerald would sing a note and this sound would shatter a glass. These are both illustrations of the use of resonance—in these examples, it dissolves the structures. When applied in this manner, the resonance eradicates unwanted invaders from the body. Such use of sound can be very effective in dealing with the resonant frequency of a bacteria or virus that's attacking the body. In these situations, the frequency of a specific invader is projected to that pathogen with enough sound energy (called amplitude) present that it shatters like a glass.

This approach to sound healing is not as widespread as the first, which focuses on using frequencies to enhance the natural, healthy resonance in order to create health. It is, nevertheless, an equally important consideration for the application of sound. In addition, sometimes the two are applied together, with one sound enhancing the healthy frequency of an organ, for example, while the other is disturbing the field being generated by an invading virus. Sometimes the two frequencies are one: While the healthy resonance of an organ is strengthened, the invading virus (or whatever) becomes weakened and is destroyed.

Please keep both of these approaches in mind as we continue our journey into the remarkable world of sound healing.

CYMATICS

If sound has such great power—the ability to change molecules, for instance—and is indeed the original creative force, then where's the proof of this claim? You would think that if we were really dealing with such a great energy, there would at least be some data to corroborate this ability of sound . . . and indeed there is.

People have known about resonance for hundreds, if not thousands, of years (perhaps back to Joshua's era!). In modern times, architects, for example, have to know about resonance when they design buildings so that the structures don't begin to vibrate in the wind and collapse.

Perhaps the most important figure in the field of sound with regard to demonstrating sound's effects was a visionary Swiss medical doctor named Hans Jenny. Dr. Jenny's seminal work, entitled *Cymatics* (derived from the Greek for "waveform"), shows the effects of sound waves on many different types of material, including pastes, liquids, and plastics. Dr. Jenny placed these substances on a steel plate; vibrated the plate with a crystal oscillator, which produces an exact frequency; and then photographed the effects. Among the many different shapes he captured were those of liquid plastic (a material like fluid Silly Putty), which formed itself into an object resembling a sea anemone; lycopodium dust (a material like talcum power), which became a shape akin to the cells of the body; and water, which took on many extraordinary geometric forms.

Dr. Jenny's work demonstrates positive proof of the amazing power of sound to create form. While the structures and objects created aren't living creatures, many of them certainly look as if they were. One can almost imagine that with a divine sound coming from a sacred source, in the beginning the "Word" could indeed create life.

The work of Dr. Jenny, who died in 1972, has been carried on by several people in the 21st century, including Alexander Lauterwasser of Germany and John Reid of England. The following are two photos created by Erik Larson of Reid's CymaScope demonstrating the images that water on a steel plate created when exposed to two different frequencies.

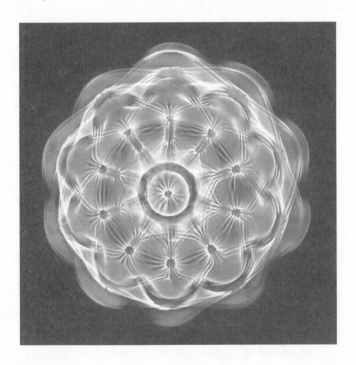

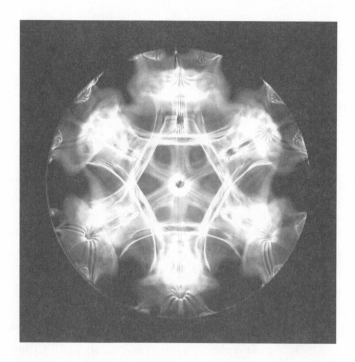

I'd like to share the words of my renowned colleague Vickie Dodd with you on the subject of the ability of sound to affect the physical body. Years ago, when we were discussing cymatics and how sound could so readily create different shapes in water, she laughed and said, "Well, my goodness, do you realize how much of our bodies is composed of water and how easy it is for sound to affect it? We're just big walking bags of water that sound can shift and change at any time."

ENTRAINMENT

Another important principle of vibration is entrainment—considered to be a subcategory of resonance. Entrainment is a phenomenon of sound in which the powerful vibrations of one object actually change those of another, causing this second object to lock in step or synchronize with the first.

We undergo entrainment frequently, shifting and changing with the different external vibrations we're exposed to. We also experience it all the time with respect to our internal rhythms. Our heart and breathing rates and brain-wave activity all entrain with one another. If you want to experience this immediately, simply take a few deep, long breaths. By slowing down your respiration in this manner, you're also moderating your heart rate and brain waves. Conversely, when you slow down your brain waves, you also decrease your heart and respiration rates.

BRAIN WAVES

Our brains pulsate and vibrate, producing electromagnetic frequencies that can be measured, just like sound, in cycles per second (or Hz). In addition, there are specific sound frequencies that influence our brain waves! Different brain-wave activity has been correlated with a specific spectrum of frequencies, known as brain-wave states, going from about .5 Hz to 20 Hz:

- **Beta waves** (14–20 Hz) are found in our normal waking state of consciousness, and are present when our focus of attention is on activities of the external world.

- **Alpha waves** (8–13 Hz) occur when we daydream and are often associated with a state of meditation. Alpha waves become stronger and more regular when our eyes are closed.

- **Theta waves** (4–7 Hz) are found in states of high creativity and have been equated with levels of consciousness found in much shamanic work. Theta waves also occur in states of deep meditation and sleep.

- **Delta waves** (.5–3 Hz) occur in states of deep sleep or unconsciousness. Some of the newer brain-wave work indicates that deep meditation produces delta waves in conscious individuals.

Two other delineations of brain-wave activity have been noted by some researchers:

- **High beta waves** (20–30 Hz) are associated with hyperactivity and some types of anxiety.

- **Gamma waves** (30–80+ Hz) have been found in seasoned meditators. Gamma waves seem to indicate bursts of precognition or high-level information processing, such as a sudden integration of ideas or experiences.

SONIC ENTRAINMENT

Most of the frequency bandwidths are very slow moving and fall just under our ability to distinguish them as individual notes. Sounds below our threshold of hearing are known as extremely low frequencies or ELFs. As previously stated, they may also be referred to as *infrasound.* While we can't usually hear them as single tones, we can actually perceive them as a kind of "wah-wah" sound. These brain-wave frequencies are measured in the same bandwidth as sound—in cycles per second (Hz). It has been demonstrated that specific sonic frequencies can actually affect our brain waves. Robert Monroe and the Monroe Institute did much of the pioneering research on this topic.

The technology to affect and change brain-wave frequencies has many names, but it's generically known as *sonic entrainment,* a term I first used in the mid-1980s to describe this phenomenon in a paper I presented for the International Society for Music Medicine. The basic principle for creating sonic entrainment is quite simple: If you take one frequency and put it in one ear and then take another frequency and put it in the other, the predominant lobes of the brain will resonate to a new frequency, which is the difference between the first two. In other words, if you put a frequency of 104 Hz in one ear and a frequency of 100 Hz in the other ear, the brain will entrain (or lock in step) with a frequency of 4 Hz, the difference between 104 and 100.

An additional name for this phenomenon is a "binaural beat frequency." Another example of this would be if you put 261 Hz in one ear and 251 Hz in the other, in which case you'd get an entrainment frequency of 10 Hz (261 − 251 = 10). You can use the difference between almost any two frequencies, as long as they're within the bandwidth of brain-wave activity (.5 Hz to 20 Hz), and you'll get some results.

It's important to understand that while there's a correlation between sonic entrainment frequencies and brain-wave activity, there isn't necessarily an exact one-to-one relationship between these resonances and the responses of the people receiving them. For example, if the difference between sonic entrainment frequencies is 4 cycles per second, not everyone will manifest brain-wave activity that matches 4 Hz. In addition, some people are going to be more susceptible than others. Not everyone is going to be affected in the same way. It's quite possible that some people, in fact, *won't* be affected. Nevertheless, the ability of sound to influence our brain waves is an important phenomenon.

Regarding sonic entrainment, please be aware that the electromagnetic frequencies of the brain aren't the same as those of its cellular structure. It's truly apples and oranges—two different things. Sound waves seem to be able to affect our brain waves and nervous system, but that's not the same as frequencies affecting the molecular structure of the brain.

Sonic entrainment continues to gain merit in the field of sound healing. Monroe found that not only did a person's brain waves entrain to the difference in frequencies, but the left and right cerebral hemispheres also synchronized as well, creating a balance. Monroe found this technology extremely effective for a variety of different activities, from enhancing deep relaxation and meditation to stimulating and increasing learning. Depending upon the frequencies used, sonic entrainment has many varied applications, including stress reduction, sleep enhancement, sharpened mental clarity, and deep introspective thinking—all of which have healing potential.

WHAT IS HEALING?

Before we continue any further, it's important that we have a mutual understanding of what's meant by *healing,* as this word can indicate many different things to many different people. For our purposes, we'll consult *The American Heritage Dictionary,* which says that the word *heal*—and its verbal relations *healed, healing,* and *heals*—means:

1. To restore to health or soundness; cure
2. To set right; repair
3. To restore (a person) to spiritual wholeness

It then adds: "To become whole and sound; return to health." I personally like this last addendum the best simply because it uses the words *sound* and *health* in the same sentence. If we can agree on this definition, then we have a common understanding—sound healing is the ability of sound to repair aspects of ourselves that are out of alignment (and need repair), as well as to restore us to spiritual wholeness.

To many people, the term *sound healing* is synonymous with the use of sound to relax and, therefore, to relieve stress. Almost everyone is familiar with the quote by English playwright William Congreve: "Music hath charms to soothe the savage breast." Twenty-five years ago, if I mentioned sound healing, the nearly universal response I'd receive had something to do with the ability of sound to soothe and calm. There's no doubt that this *is* an important and powerful aspect of sound; however, the ability to make whole, to repair, and to return to health requires another understanding of sound for healing: the power to rearrange molecules.

In February 1988, the Science section of *The New York Times* contained the following headline: "Sound Is Shaped Into a Dazzling Tool With Many Uses." The article went on to state: "The beams can make, break or rearrange molecules, control the crystalline structure of matter and even levitate objects or blobs of liquid." In other words, sound is not just an energy that enters our ears and our brains, allowing us to experience the sensation of hearing; it also has the ability to go into our cellular structure and rearrange our molecules. Awareness of this extraordinary quality is necessary for us to recognize the true power of sound to heal.

Thus, for a true understanding of this power, we must include the complete quote from William Congreve:

Music hath charms to soothe the savage breast,
To soften rocks, or bend a knotted oak [boldface is mine].

Once again, to repeat, we are talking about an energy that not only enters our ears and our brains and is able to affect our nervous system, but which also goes into our cellular structure and has the ability to rearrange our molecules. Congreve may have been speaking metaphorically, but he was quite accurate—except, of course, he should have been talking about sound and not music.

SOUND VS. MUSIC

No doubt you're asking yourself, *What is this author talking about?* Most of us think of sound and music as being the same thing, but it's important for our purposes to highlight the difference between them. Simply put, when you hear a symphony or band, what's produced is music—it's usually a complex and orderly arrangement of different sounds. When a tree falls in the forest and you hear it crash to the ground, that's sound; very few people would consider it to be music.

I make this distinction because many times the sounds that are used in healing aren't necessarily very musical. Sometimes they're quite soothing and melodic, but many times they're not. It's important for anyone exploring the arena of sound healing to realize that audible vibrations used for healing may not always have musical tones. They may, in fact, have the opposite. You might be expecting some harmonious sound, but instead it's quite possible that you experience something more akin to hearing the hum of a refrigerator or the buzz of a fan. For most people, this isn't music—it might, however, be quite healing.

Again, I make this distinction based on my own need to separate sound and music. Conceptually, all sound is music, but in truth I think that there are few of you reading this who'd think that the sound of a tree crashing in the woods or a piece of chalk grating on a blackboard is very musical. More realistically, all music is sound, but not vice versa: Not all sound is music. I think that Julie Andrews (courtesy of Rogers & Hammerstein) got it right when she sang "The Sound of Music."

Please be aware that when I discuss sound, I'll usually be talking about single tones that don't change or modulate with all the elements that we've come to expect in music: melody, harmony, rhythm, and so forth. When I'm talking about sounds that do contain those elements (the sounds that most of us in the West consider musical), I'll use the word *music.* Of course, for some people the buzzing of a chainsaw can be a symphony, but for our purposes we'll deal with the delineation as stated.

Scientists have speculated that the original creative sound—what has been called the "big bang"—was actually an extraordinarily deep note, much slower and deeper than anything that could possibly be heard. Some have referred to this as the "cosmic hum." We may never know what this sound was really like or whether it was the original "Word" of creation— the vibration that manifested the universe from its resonance. But it's yet another indication of the significance of our first secret: Everything is vibration. Not only is everything in a state of vibration, but ultimately everything *came from* vibration.

Let's now continue on our journey with an exercise that's designed to help you experience the importance of sound in your life.

••• Exercise 1 •••

We live in a world of sound. The aim of this exercise to remind you of that fact and allow you to establish a relationship with the sound in your surrounding environment.

Hearing is the very first sense to be activated in us, even before we're born, and it's the last to leave us once we pass on. We actually become sensitive to sound as early as the ninth week in utero. According to those who've had a near-death experience, we're able to perceive sounds even after our breathing and heartbeat have stopped.

Our perception of the world and our definition of reality comes from our senses. When we enhance our ability to use any one of them, it actually changes the way that we perceive the world and reality.

Find a relatively quiet place where you won't be disturbed. Sit comfortably in a chair. Look around and observe the different components of this space as you may perceive them. Now close your eyes. Instead of using your eyes and your sense of sight to receive, encode, and explore information from the outside world, utilize your ears and your sense of hearing. Is there a difference? What do you notice? Become aware of all the subtle nuances of sound that may be present. Do you hear your refrigerator humming or the clock ticking? Is there a dog barking on your street? Do you hear the neighbors' TV or perhaps their lawn mower?

Be as still as you can. Become aware of your breath. The quieter you become, the more conscious you'll be of the myriad different sounds in your environment. The more you focus on and become aware of them, the more this awareness will change the information you receive about your surroundings and your world. As you practice this exercise, slowly begin to shift your focus of awareness from the sounds nearest you to those farthest away. What can you hear off in the distance? Are you able to visualize or feel the energy of whatever it is that you're hearing?

Now, bring your focus of sonic awareness back to the sounds of the space you're sitting in. Practice this form of deep listening and become aware of the changes that occur within your consciousness through this exercise.

Note: If you like, you can repeat this exercise, as well as the others in this book, on a daily basis. While this isn't necessary, daily repetition will provide beneficial results. Each time you practice the exercises, they'll probably be a little different and will further open you up to the extraordinary world of sound.

• • ● • •

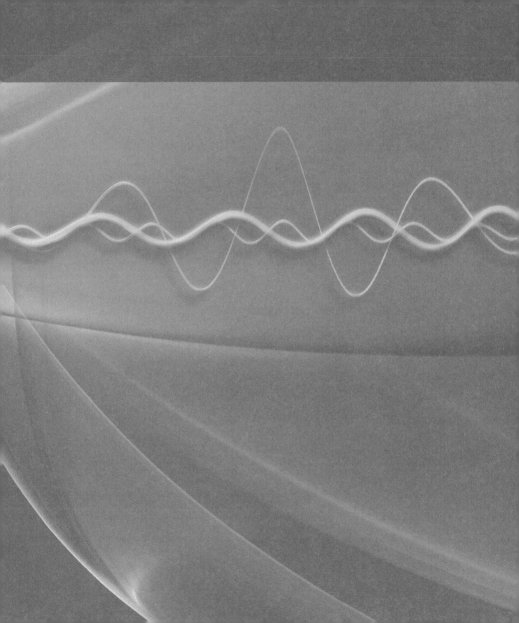

Secret 2

Intent
Is
Powerful

Before we go into exploring this next secret, I must tell you a story. It happened almost 20 years ago, and it molded the foundation of my current belief system about sound healing. Thus, it's important that I share it with you.

I was sitting at my computer working on my first book. I like to say that this was so long ago that my computer still used DOS (if you're not old enough to remember what that is, know that it was a while ago). I'd spent years collecting an extremely large amount of information about systems that used sound and music for healing, and at the time I was compiling it all in a book. (As I mentioned in the Preface, I had at one point in my life collected an encyclopedic amount of information—this was at that point.) I had a stack of papers that was literally two feet high, and it was composed of nothing more (or less) than various systems that used different frequencies and tones for healing. It was all very fascinating . . . and it was all very frustrating because nothing correlated. There was nothing consistent about any of the information. I'd collected data from hundreds of different sources, and little of it was in agreement.

Scientist A would use a particular frequency for one organ. Scientist B would use a completely different one for the same organ. Both scientists would claim success. Spiritual Master L would use a specific mantra to achieve one effect. Spiritual Master M would use a different mantra for the same result. Both masters would also claim success.

I had pages and pages of different systems, and nothing matched. It made no sense to my scientific and logical "left-brained" background. If the information that I just shared with you in the last chapter was true, then surely there would be some similarity between the different systems. Yet there wasn't. On and on, page after page, I found different sounds being used, apparently very successfully, to treat different conditions and achieve different states of being. How could this be?

I remember sitting with my head in my hands in a condition of intellectual angst, staring at the computer screen, trying to make sense of it all. And then something happened that changed my life: I distinctly became aware of an inner voice that said, *It is not only the frequency of the sound that creates its effect, but also the intention of the user.* I then wrote down this formula: *Frequency + Intent = Healing.* After that, my life was different and everything made sense.

FREQUENCY + INTENT = HEALING

What does this mean? We've already discussed the essence of *frequency.* It's the measurement of sound in cycles per second and can be, from my understanding, the nature of the physical aspect of sound. *Healing* we've already defined as having to do with making something whole. But what is meant by *intent?*

Intent (also called "intention") certainly wasn't a new concept to me back all those years ago. I'd made reference to it many times in my writings. I'd simply never put it together in a formula in the way I did at that moment. Intent is the energy behind the sound. It's the consciousness we have when making the sound, which is then encoded upon it, travels on it, and ultimately is received by the person listening to it.

It finally all made sense. One person could make a sound with a certain intention, and that would be the outcome of the sound. Another person could make the same sound with a different intent, and it would have a very different outcome. Many of us have had things like this happen at times in our lives.

For example, you may be at a party and see someone whom you have some difficulty with. This person remarks, "Lovely to see you," and you feel like cringing. The words (analogous to the frequency) may have said one thing, but the intent, and ultimately the outcome of the sound, was quite another.

When I first devised my formula (and the other modifications I'll share with you shortly), I thought that I'd made a very important discovery. In truth, as I began to examine the validity of this formula, I found that while I had indeed put those words *Frequency + Intent = Healing* together, the elements of this formula had been used in almost every spiritual tradition that utilized sound for any purpose, from healing to communing with the gods to making the crops grow. However, the importance of intent was an explanation that was missing from the understanding of so many of the modern scientists who were perceiving sound simply as frequency and nothing more.

At that time, and for several years afterward, I made a point of attempting to bring awareness of intent to as many scientists, medical doctors, and others who were focused on researching the use of sound for healing as I could. Whenever I was doing a presentation at a conference, or somehow in the company of a renowned researcher (usually an M.D. or a Ph.D.), I would ask him or her: "Have you ever considered the importance of intention?" If I got a reply at all (instead of simply being ignored by whomever I was addressing, or looked at as though I were a man from outer space), the answer was usually a simple but profoundly uninterested *No.*

How times have changed! Now I can watch specials on PBS about the power of intention. Now I'm able to freely talk about this subject matter. Now I can discuss sound healing and some people are able to think beyond that first line of "Music hath charms to soothe the savage breast." They may even understand that the world is indeed sound . . . they may even understand about intent.

KINESIOLOGY

One of the many difficulties I first encountered in my campaign to awaken awareness of intention was quite simply that intent was not a very measurable commodity. It was easy to gauge different aspects of sound, from its frequency to its amplitude (loudness) to the shape of its waveform. But how do you measure intention?

One way to do so is with applied kinesiology, a method of testing the strength of our muscles. (For the sake of simplicity, in this book I'll refer to *applied kinesiology* as "kinesiology.") Kinesiology has become so popular that many holistic-health practitioners, from chiropractors to acupuncturists, use it in their work. It's fast, it's easy to use, and the results nearly always align with solid, scientific verification if the practitioner knows what he or she is doing.

If you haven't heard of kinesiology, it's very simple. Some aspect of the body (the exact mechanism has yet to be determined— somewhat like acupuncture) responds to external input in such a way that those stimuli that are beneficial to us (this could be anything from food to herbs to music) cause our muscles to become strong. If a kinesiologist presses on a muscle (for example, the deltoid muscle of an outstretched arm of someone being tested) while that person holds something beneficial such as a piece of fresh fruit, it will be difficult for the practitioner to push the patient's arm down. However, if that individual holds something that's toxic, such as a cigarette, his or her muscles will become weakened and it will be easy to push the arm down. It's quite mysterious and fascinating if you've never encountered kinesiology before.

It's possible to test both sound and intention in this manner, as well as to demonstrate that not only do we respond differently to different sounds, but to different intentions as well. There have been many experiments documenting this. Some practitioners, such as John Diamond, M.D., have even named this force "life energy" and have done much work demonstrating its power in music.

An Experiment with Kinesiology and Intent

Perhaps my favorite experiment occurred many years ago and for me best illustrates the phenomenon of the power of intent. In this investigation, researchers went to the beach to record the sound of the ocean on a cassette recorder. First, they recorded the sound of the ocean by itself. Next, they assembled a group of meditators at the beach and asked them to silently meditate on peace and love while the sounds of the ocean were being recorded on a different cassette tape. Finally, they instructed this same group of people to think about things that made them angry and fearful. They recorded this ocean sound as well on a third cassette tape.

Now, sonically these were all the same sounds. You couldn't tell them apart. They were labeled with nondescriptive names such as *X*, *Y*, and *Z* so that the kinesiology practitioner didn't know which particular recording was playing while the subjects' arms were tested. The results of this experiment were very interesting:

1. First, the sounds of the natural ocean caused people to test strong. You would think that this would be the case—and it was. The sounds of nature are healing.

2. Second, the recording when the participants meditated on peace and love actually made those tested even stronger than the first sounds had made them—their arms were "rock solid."

3. Finally, the ocean sounds recorded when the participants were thinking of anger and fear made the arms of those tested "weak as a kitten."

This is just one example out of many kinesiology demonstrations that show how the power of intention can affect us.

AN EXPERIENCE WITH SOUND AND INTENT

As I mentioned in the beginning of this chapter, I come from a scientific background. Despite the fact that I sometimes hear guiding voices or experience other nonscientific phenomena, I'm by nature a skeptic. Thus, when I first encountered kinesiology, I was rather dubious of the results. I knew that if practitioners had an agenda to prove, they could do it. If the tester were adept enough, he or she could look at someone the wrong way and the person would test weak. Because of this, there isn't much objectivity with kinesiology. And although I've also seen and experienced skilled practitioners demonstrate remarkable and verifiable results, I still remain a skeptic.

One time I'd been working with someone who'd been demonstrating the power of sound and kinesiology to me. When this person realized my skepticism, he did a little experiment with me that didn't involve kinesiology, but nevertheless convinced me of the power of intent and sound to actually create a physical response. To begin, he put on a record album (this experience obviously occurred a long time ago when flat, thin discs with grooves in them, called LPs, were the mode of listening) and simply asked me to check myself out and notice my heartbeat and respiration. Was I breathing slowly or rapidly? Was my breath shallow or deep? How was my heart beating? Was my pulse fast or slow? I observed myself as I listened to the music and noted my response. He then put on another album, and I was again asked to check myself out as I listened to it.

This second album sounded as if it were exactly the same piece of music as the first. And it was—it featured the identical musical composition with the same orchestra. The only difference was the conductor.

I was amazed that my personal reactions were so totally different for each experience. With the first recording, I'd been relaxed, breathing slowly and deeply. My heartbeat was calm and steady. With the second, I tensed up, my breathing sped up and was shallower, and my heartbeat also became faster and more erratic. What was going on? I was having a physical reaction to sounds that were basically the same! Then the answer was revealed.

The first conductor, I was told, was a man attuned to the flow of the universe—what one might call a Zen of now. He generated peace and harmony whenever he conducted. The second conductor was a rigid perfectionist who apparently terrified his orchestra whenever he picked up the baton. This energy was obviously transmitted in the music. I was told this after I'd noted and described my experience with the different record albums.

One of my great understandings is simply this: You can read and cogitate about sound all you want, but until you've experienced something that demonstrates what you've read, then it's not true for you. I still adhere to this understanding. That day, experiencing the difference between the effects of recordings of the same music, was further validation of this concept of "life energy" and the power of intention. Our consciousness has the ability to "ride" on the sound and affect how it's received.

MASARU EMOTO

Recently the important work of Japanese scientist Masaru Emoto has reached mainstream consciousness through his many books, including *Messages from Water.* Dr. Emoto began experimenting with water, collecting samples from throughout the world, freezing them, and then photographing them using a special "dark-field" microscope.

His first photographs showed that natural water, such as that from a healthy spring, created an image that looked very much like a snowflake, while polluted water formed an image resembling mud. Dr. Emoto then began experimenting with different sounds to see their effects. The results were very similar: Certain genres of music, such as classical and New Age, created extraordinary geometric snowflake-like images, while others, such as heavy metal, created mudlike images. He continued his experimentation by taping words on bottles of distilled water to see what would happen. The results were startling: Words such as *Thank You!* created the snowflake shapes; phrases such as *You make me sick!* created mud. These later experiments demonstrate the power of intention or consciousness to affect physical matter.

For me, the most dramatic demonstration of Dr. Emoto's work involved polluted water from the Fujiwara Dam in Japan. This water, when first photographed, looked like mud. It was then chanted and prayed over by a priest for an hour. When it was photographed again, the water resembled snowflakes! These images clearly showed the power of *Frequency + Intent* to affect physical structure.

Our bodies are composed of at least 75 percent water. If a chanting priest can change the mudlike vibrations of polluted water into the snowflake-like vibrations of clean water, it really makes us realize the power of sound and consciousness to heal not only our physical bodies, but this entire planet.

What follows are two photographs of Dr. Emoto's work. The first shows the mudlike image of the water from the Fujiwara Dam before it was chanted over; the second, the same water after it had been chanted over.

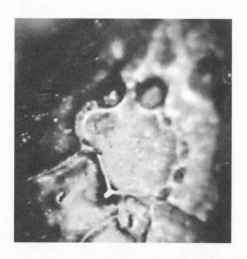

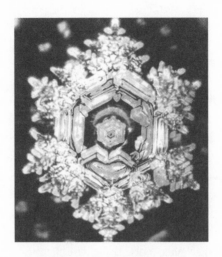

VOCALIZATION + VISUALIZATION = MANIFESTATION

The ability of consciousness to be encoded upon sound waves is an extremely important phenomenon of sound healing—a secret we really need to embrace. Hence, in addition to my formula *Frequency + Intent = Healing*, one can also use *Vocalization + Visualization = Manifestation*. The meaning of the latter is similar to that of the former, except that here we have a vocalized sound (created by someone using their voice) plus visualization (the process of imagining something or someone) creating manifestation (the actual outcome). For example, someone might chant a mantra to invoke a specific deity while also visualizing this divine being. The result would be a manifestation of the energy of this higher power.

This phenomenon of using *Vocalization* and *Visualization* in order to create *Manifestation* is a practice that many who engage with sacred sound, and in particular those who chant mantras, have experienced. The power is undeniable. The application of this formula may in fact be observed in almost every sacred path that employs sound. When praying aloud and chanting, spiritual adepts will invoke and visualize specific energies or deities and then experience them. Those practitioners of the Tibetan tradition are perhaps among the most proficient at this—in their meditation, the technology of visualization is a skill that they spend a great deal of time developing. These visualizations, when coupled with their mantra chanting, create extraordinary effects.

SOUND + BELIEF = OUTCOME

One last formula I recently created was influenced by the work of Gregg Braden, an esteemed colleague. His book *The Isaiah Effect* focuses on the power of feeling as an important amplifier for the manifestation of prayer. According to Gregg, as well as researchers at the Institute of HeartMath, the energy of emotion—when it's felt and generated from within—creates a coherent resonant electromagnetic field between the heart and the brain that's much greater than that generated by the brain itself. Feeling may, therefore, be one of the major keys to manifesting prayer.

In addition, in his book *The Divine Matrix,* Gregg also emphasizes the importance and power of belief in the creation of reality. He investigates the new quantum understanding of our ability, as scientists have observed experimentally, to influence the state of an electron, transforming it from a wave to a particle. There's no longer simply an onlooker watching an experiment. The mere act of observation actually influences the outcome. It would be more accurate that this observer now be called a *participant,* since he or she is engaged not only in the experiment, but in the co-creation of reality as well. Gregg suggests that in such circumstances belief is the code that translates invisible energy (waves) into visible matter (particles).

This prompted me to create yet a third formula to describe the relationship between sound and consciousness and its ability to change reality, which is perhaps the easiest of all to understand. It is this: *Sound + Belief = Outcome.*

The relationship between the body and mind has been extensively documented in recent years. Our bodies can influence our minds, and vice versa. Thus, our thoughts, beliefs, intention, feelings, consciousness—whatever you'd like to call it—can affect us physically. The placebo effect has demonstrated that people can take sugar pills with the understanding that they're actual pharmaceutical drugs and report experiencing the specific effects of the supposed drug. While most people cite that 30 percent of those tested are subject to the placebo effect, new research seems to indicate that the actual percentage is much higher—up to 80 percent under certain conditions.

The New England Journal of Medicine has even reported the results of a very well-designed study at a Houston VA hospital. Doctors performed arthroscopic knee surgery on one group of patients with arthritis, scraping and rinsing their knee joints. In another group, the doctors made small cuts in the patients' knees to mimic the incisions of a real operation and then bandaged them up. The pain relief reported by the two groups was identical. What all this means is still speculative, although the implications are quite astounding: It does seem to indicate that there's an important and, for the most part, unexplored relationship between our thoughts/feelings/belief/intentions and the ability of our bodies to respond to treatment.

I'd like to suggest, once again, that indeed *Frequency + Intent = Healing;* and that it's one of the most important of the 7 Secrets of Sound Healing, for it may provide an explanation of the extraordinary variety of approaches, frequencies, and sounds that seems to manifest positive and life-affirming changes for people.

••• Exercise 2 •••

Intent influences and affects the different sounds you project and receive. This exercise will assist you in increasing your awareness of its power.

Think back to a time when you may have experienced an aspect of the power of intent as it was encoded upon sound. As I mentioned in this chapter, perhaps there was an occasion at a party or a similar event when you saw someone you had issues with who smiled at you, came up to you, and said something quite nice. However, instead of feeling what his or her words communicated, you sensed a hidden undercurrent of negativity. The individual's sound (the frequency) indicated one thing, but the intention that you picked up was quite different.

Find someone who's willing to work with you for a similar experiment, and say something kind to him or her, such as "I love you" (or whatever is appropriate), while you're projecting some sort of negative intent—anger, for example. Then try repeating the same thing while you're actually projecting this vibration of kindness. Ask the other person if he or she can feel a difference; then have him or her try the same thing on you and determine if *you* can. Make a note about any changes in the vocal tone you may have heard as you projected a different intent onto the same words.

It's actually very difficult to project intention without this being reflected in the sound of your voice. Tone most often expresses feeling and, very frequently, your intent. The odds are that you'll be able to immediately discern a shift in the energy when projecting and receiving different intentions. More often than not, you'll also be able to detect a change in tone. Please be sure that you end with a positive and kind intent—you don't want anyone walking away with negative energy!

· • ● • ·

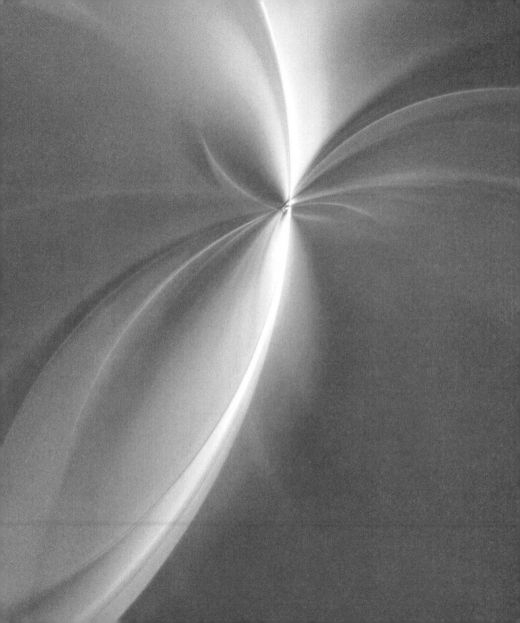

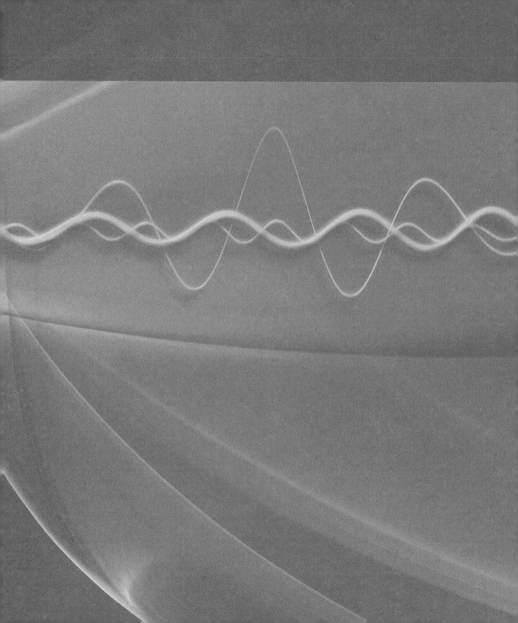

Secret 3

We Are All
Unique
Vibratory
Beings

The next secret is this: We are all unique vibratory beings. This means that we're all individuals, and what works for one person may not work for another.

As Secret 1 indicates, everything is vibration. Our vibratory rates aren't the same and in fact might be quite distinct for each of us. They may only vary slightly, but they *are* different. Indeed, the ability to modulate frequencies and shift vibrations may be one of the most extraordinary benefits of using sound as a transformative modality.

During workshops and lectures, I like to take a poll that's related to this secret. I ask, "Is anyone here allergic to penicillin?" Then I look around at the raised hands and nod my head, because usually anywhere from 10 to 20 percent of the people in the room are allergic to this antibiotic. I use this as a metaphor for us all being unique vibratory beings.

I continue: "Well, if everything in the universe is in a state of vibration and is a waveform, this includes pharmaceuticals. Therefore, there's a frequency for penicillin. And for about 80 percent of you, this frequency will heal you under the right circumstances; but for about 20 percent of you, it will be toxic. Now, how could this be true if we were all vibrating at the same frequency?"

I use penicillin as an example, but I could easily refer to some other substance that provides the same results, showing that not everything is going to affect everybody in the same way. I believe that most of us are aware of this intuitively—a knowing that has manifested in sayings such as "Different strokes for different folks" or "One man's meat is another man's poison." This is certainly common sense, but sometimes we forget it—especially when listening to supposed experts who tell us differently.

MUSIC AND THE PSYCHE

Back in the 1930s, a man by the name of Carl Seashore, the author of *Psychology of Music,* began to study how music affects the psyche of different people. (Here, again, I'm using "music" to mean specific compositions that are considered musical to our Western ears.) Back then, Seashore and others didn't have medical equipment to hook people up to in order to check their brain waves or other anatomical functions and determine how they were being affected. Instead, they simply gave those being tested questionnaires. Called "semantic differentials," these surveys allowed people to rate music. This may seem fairly primitive in our modern computer age, but it was quite effective.

I remember studying this work and being impressed because it showed that there was no major consensus on anything! Often about 40 percent of the people tested would really like one piece of music, while another 40 percent would strongly *dis*like it. The last 20 percent were neutral and had no preference. The musical selection that elicited the most agreement from those tested was John Philip Sousa's "The Stars and Stripes Forever," but even this piece only garnered positive responses from about 70 percent of the people. The majority found Sousa's marching song to be stimulating and uplifting; however, 20 percent found it sad and depressing, and the remaining 10 percent claimed either not to be affected by it or not to care one way or the other.

That was the piece of music the most people agreed upon— only 70 percent! That's probably a good statistic to work with in terms of the effects of music (and also sound) on the body, mind, and spirit. Everyone is going to be a little different, and if you can get a 70 percent response with anything—whether it's a pharmaceutical drug or a frequency—you're doing quite well. Thus, with regard to finding a frequency that will work for everyone, there may be a generic sound that creates a positive response from 70 percent of the people. I doubt you'll find anything more effective than that.

It's simply not my experience that we all vibrate to the same frequency, particularly in our physical bodies. In the 1980s, Dr. Peter Guy Manners, a British osteopath who had been working with sound for more than 20 years, made a statement in a lecture that seemed rather important. He talked about the difference in the vibrational rates of people and suggested that these differences could be the reason why transplanted organs might be rejected.

There's little hard data on this subject, but it's an interesting point of conjecture—especially when dealing with the topic of vibrational medicine. There are numerous stories about how people who've received donated organs can develop tastes for food as well as other characteristics that were exhibited by the donors. This seems to indicate some sort of vibrational resonance inherent in the organ and transmitted to its recipient.

TIME AND CIRCUMSTANCE

Other factors besides the particular resonance of a person also influence the sound's specific effects. Time and circumstance may be very important as far as what sounds are most effective for us, just as they may also indicate which music may be most beneficial for our healing.

Having been in this field for a long time, I've seen many different varieties declared to be "the" healing music. Conversely, I've seen many different genres denounced as the opposite. This is nonsense. Any type, depending on the time, place, and needs of the individual, can be healing.

Let me illustrate this point. I used to live in the mountains outside of Boulder, Colorado, in an isolated environment where the elevation was over 9,000 feet. Living so high up provided many challenges, including the necessity of working and teaching in Boulder, which was nearly a mile in altitude below my mountain home, as well as being an hour's drive away.

The main road from the mountains down to Boulder is two lanes and at times as winding as a pretzel. It's also extremely dangerous to travel on because weather conditions can change dramatically as you go up in elevation.

It was challenging! The road would be icy. There would be whiteouts. And if by chance someone drove off the road— well, sometimes the drop would be lethal. Navigating the canyon wasn't something that anyone undertook lightly, especially during inclement weather. There would be many times when I'd finish teaching late at night and I'd encounter exactly these conditions as I was going home, driving from moderate weather into a snowstorm.

Frequently, when driving down the canyon during the day, I'd play gentle and relaxing music. I was awake. Visibility was good. I could sit back and have a pleasant drive, and it would be great.

But if I listened to the same music late at night when I was tired, I found that it made me drowsy and ill equipped to handle the drive—especially when going into a blizzard. The same music that had been stress reducing and healing under one set of conditions was now dangerous under another. I'd usually put on very fast-paced music and turn it up quite loud. The combination of these two factors created a sonic-caffeine effect that was useful in terms of keeping me alert and allowing me to drive in adverse weather conditions.

Please remember—this is what worked for me. I use it as an example to illustrate how the same music can affect someone differently depending upon the time and the circumstances. Many people may relate to my experience of using various types of music to drive the canyon—but not everyone. Some folks play calm and slow music to stay alert and centered. Once again, this is because we're all unique vibratory beings.

I often create music that's useful for relaxation and stress reduction. Sometimes it's so powerful that I won't listen to it in a car; I'll only do so while lying down.

Once, after I'd created and produced one of these recordings, I encountered a gentleman who was a truck driver. He was, to my recollection, the first person who actually purchased that particular recording. I remember that I saw him about a month afterward, and he thanked me for creating such a profound and powerful sound experience. I gratefully acknowledged his thanks and asked him how he'd used the recording.

"Oh," he replied, "it was what kept me going when I did my East Coast–West Coast trips."

I did a double take and interjected, "But you're not supposed to use it when you drive!"

The gentleman shrugged his shoulders and said, "Works for me."

Thus, whether it's chakra resonance or truck driving, I'd like to suggest that we simply can't make the assumption that any particular sound or music is going to affect everyone in the same way. Not only are we all unique vibratory beings, but the circumstances and conditions under which we listen to these sounds will also be quite distinct.

MAGIC FREQUENCIES

It's important to be aware that we're all unique vibratory beings and different sounds affect us all very differently because of the many claims that have emerged about there being magic frequencies.

Magic frequency is a term for a "sonic cure-all" that doesn't exist. Ever since I first began my journey into exploring the uses of sound and music for healing more than 25 years ago, I've continually encountered people who were searching for specific frequencies that would heal and transform everyone. Sometimes it was the frequency for a particular body part, such as the liver or the heart. Occasionally, it was for a particular emotion, such as love or hate. Sometimes it was for a condition, such as male sexual stimulation (we're talking about sonic Viagra here!), asthma, or even cancer.

Over the years, this trend hasn't changed. The more people learn about the power of sound to heal and transform, the more they're interested in discovering and using an individual frequency to treat a specific problem, enhance a particular organ, or do some other extraordinary thing. Who can blame them? The idea makes sense: If everything is vibration, then why *wouldn't* there be an overall vibration that could be used to cure everyone?

As I said, I call these panaceas that people are searching for *magic frequencies.* It reminds me of the Walt Disney movie *Dumbo,* where the young elephant is given a "magic" feather that enables him to fly. At the end of the film, we learn that there's nothing special about the feather; it was simply Dumbo's belief in the object that created the flying phenomenon. Disney may have been one of the first to tap into the extraordinary power of the placebo effect!

Another reason why I call these frequencies "magic" is because if they exist, I don't think that anyone has found them yet. I've certainly encountered numerous people who *claim* that they have. And of course, if you've come across one frequency that has a specific healing purpose, then often you've found others as well—usually dozens, sometimes hundreds or even thousands of them. I know people who have books filled with such magic frequencies.

I, in fact, have been one of these people. I probably have one of the larger collections of such frequencies on the planet, found in that stack of papers I previously mentioned, which led me to the creation of the *Frequency + Intent = Healing* formula. A difference, perhaps, is that I didn't actually discover any of these frequencies myself, and thus don't have any attachment to them. In addition, recall that I had the experience where I found that these different frequencies simply had no compatibility with one another. I'd gathered all of them together and then sat there scratching my head, trying to make sense of everything, until the formula applying both frequency and intent manifested for me.

At that time, I'd also been mystified that the discoverers of these different magic frequencies could all claim extraordinary success. I don't think I ever found the disclaimer WON'T WORK FOR EVERYONE attached to any of these sonic codes. Sometimes I'd meet people who'd had amazing healing experiences with these frequencies; occasionally, I'd even have them myself. On the other hand, I'd also meet people who had received frequencies that either had a negative effect or no effect whatsoever. I, too, have experienced this. It certainly makes believing in such magic frequencies difficult.

I remember a student once called me from overseas. She'd felt fine but had wanted to experience a particular form of sound healing that intrigued her. She received a treatment from a practitioner who'd been trained in one of the therapies that use magic frequencies. She told me that afterward she'd become very sick for about a week: She was nauseated and fatigued and could barely get out of bed. She'd used one of my CDs to help bring herself back into balance so that she could resume her normally healthful life. I don't know whether this student actually benefited from listening to the CD, but I *certainly* believe that she had a negative reaction to whatever frequency she received.

The student asked me what she should do, as the practitioner wanted her back for another session the next week. I suggested that perhaps she should forgo returning—going back just didn't make sense to me. But the student went anyway and called me a week later—she'd become even sicker than before; and this time, according to her, even my CD was of no use. There wasn't much I could say. Fortunately, she called again several weeks later to tell me that she'd recovered.

It's been my experience that most of the time, if a sound is good for you, you'll *feel* good. You'll have a positive reaction. You won't get sick. However, if a sound isn't right for you, you *won't* feel good after exposure to it. In fact, you may get sick and feel bad.

The occurrence of pain is rare when dealing with sound-healing frequencies—in fact, it hasn't been my personal experience. If a sound has an adverse reaction for me, I know that it's one that doesn't resonate with me and I no longer listen to it—it's that simple.

When others are listening to a recording or doing an exercise and experience some discomfort, I almost always say, "Stop listening to the CD!" or "Quit doing the exercise!" It doesn't make sense to try to resonate with a frequency that makes you feel ill. Such experiences are usually the result of therapists who believe in the concept of magic frequencies and try to encode their belief upon others: "This is the right frequency for you! Your body simply isn't used to it—just give it some time."

I share this with you in the event that as you begin to explore the world of sound, you encounter such a situation. I'm simply not a big believer in the "No pain, no gain" method of healing. I'm sure that there's some validity to it, and there may be times when such an experience is necessary. But, if possible, I try to stay away from it.

It's just common sense. If a doctor gives you a prescription and that medicine makes you ill, you would call up the physician to let him or her know. Nine times out of ten, any self-respecting M.D. will tell you to stop taking the drug. I'd highly recommend that anyone reading this book heed such advice. If you're trying a particular sound therapy that makes you sick, then try something else.

Sound is a sonic nutrient. It feeds and nourishes body, mind, and spirit. Alfred Tomatis, M.D., demonstrated that certain sounds charge our brains and our nervous systems. Our sonic appetite should, therefore, be broad and include many of the diverse aspects of the sound spectrum found throughout this planet (particularly the music from different countries and cultures)—all the various genres that are available, from jazz to classical to folk to opera to blues.

Sometimes we may hear music that's alien and strange to us and dislike it. No doubt, this is a bit like sampling a new and different food. Then our taste buds adapt, and we learn to love what we first found unusual. However, this educational process of sampling music and determining whether we like it is different from torturing ourselves by listening to sound that makes us sick. To repeat: If something affects you negatively when you hear it, turn it off! There's no magic frequency, and if there were, it certainly wouldn't make you feel bad.

Dr. Herbert Benson, the author of *The Relaxation Response,* has discussed the concept of Tibetan medicine, in which there are three components:

1. The belief of the person receiving the healing in the healer

2. The belief of the healer in the medicine

3. The relationship between the healer and person receiving the healing

The first two elements deal with "belief," which I've already discussed. The third element relates to the interaction between two people. From a Western energetic understanding, we can perceive this simply as two people being in resonance with each other.

Have you ever had the experience of going to a doctor or a therapist whom someone has recommended to you as being the "best," and your visit has suggested to you that he or she was in fact the "worst"? Regardless of the reason for your dislike, it's doubtful that you found whatever medicine this person practiced to be effective for you. This is yet another example of how difficult it would be for a magic frequency to exist—based upon Dr. Benson's principles, not everyone is going to have the same reaction.

Deb Shapiro, a renowned author, has written a wonderful book called *Your Body Speaks Your Mind,* which focuses on the interconnection between physical imbalances and our minds and emotions. In healing, Deb suggests that there are many different levels that need to be examined for treatment, and it's important that the appropriate one be dealt with. If someone has a headache, it's simple enough to take an aspirin. But if the problem is stemming from an emotional issue—perhaps a situation occurring at work or at home—or if it's due to an environmental issue, such as an allergic reaction to some food or exposure to a toxic chemical, then the aspirin won't help heal the underlying problem. It's important to get to the source—the originating cause of the issue. The same is true with using sound to heal.

Dr. Randall McClellan once related a story to me that I'd like to share with you. It describes a phenomenon that I've experienced and can attest to.

Randall had a pain in his shoulder and used a particular sound instrument to heal this condition. Sure enough, for several days the discomfort went away. Then it came back, and he used the instrument again. The pain disappeared for a few more days before returning, and he continued with the treatment in this manner.

"You know, Jonathan," he told me, "it's a bit like someone having a nail sticking through their shoe. You can put on a bandage, and it will help for a while, but until you're able to locate the nail and take it out, the condition will continue." There's much truth and wisdom in that story, and it illustrates an important point: Not everyone will always be healed by sound—or any other modality.

I've personally experienced instantaneous and permanent healing effects from sound, and I've witnessed seemingly miraculous occurrences! Sound is multidimensional and can therefore work simultaneously on many levels—physical, emotional, mental, and spiritual.

If sound can, among other things, change molecular structure, its potential regenerative power is unlimited. At the same time, I've also seen absolutely nothing occur after someone received a session of sound healing. I have no satisfying explanation for the paradox inherent in this but merely note that I've witnessed both scenarios. Whether it was simply the wrong frequency, the wrong practitioner delivering it, or the disbelief of the person on the receiving end can never be known—but nothing happened. Here again is another indication that there are no magic frequencies. We are unique vibratory beings—we may require unique vibratory medicine . . . and we may each need unique ways of receiving it.

In recent years, the awareness of sound as a healing and transformative modality has begun to infiltrate the consciousness of more and more people. As the interest increases, the search for magic frequencies also intensifies and the unproven claims made about them mount. Due to lack of knowledge and overenthusiasm on the part of some healers, more misinformation about sound frequencies is now being perpetuated.

It's important to understand the fallacy of this magic-frequency concept. By recognizing the uniqueness of our own vibratory resonance, we can better maintain awareness of the true power of sound to heal and transform, avoiding the pitfalls that come from misinformation and exaggerated claims.

THE SCHUMANN RESONANCE

An entire book could be written researching the validity of magic frequencies. Many more people are now making remarkable claims about different ones, and there are few who question this. Perhaps the most popular among these claims has to do with finding the frequency that's resonant with the earth. This is the number one magic frequency, and it may be so because it's based on an actual scientific measurement. There is, in fact, a geophysical bandwidth called the Schumann resonance. Named after physicist W. O. Schumann, who predicted it mathematically in 1952, it's the resonance of low-frequency electromagnetic waves bouncing around the cavity of the earth, which acts as an active resonant chamber.

The frequency of the Schumann resonance is said to be 7.83 Hz. However, in reality, this isn't an actual frequency at all. Rather, it's the average peak resonance of the space between the earth's surface and the ionosphere, which changes due to a number of variables, including environmental conditions—such as temperature and lightning—as well as the activity of sunspots. Thus, 7.83 Hz is merely an average, representing a waveform that's not constant, but rather fluctuates immensely.

If you do an Internet search for the Schumann resonance, you'll find more than a quarter of a million Websites that have information on this topic. You'll encounter everything from geophysical data to sites selling CDs that claim to contain the Schumann-resonance frequency and promise to do everything from enhance your IQ to give you psychic abilities. There's probably more misinformation out there about the Schumann resonance than all other magic frequencies put together.

If the "top" magic frequency isn't a static, constant tone, but is fluid and variable, it really makes you wonder about any others that are being claimed. No doubt people are experiencing profound and powerful results with these different frequencies, but this may be based more on their expectation than anything else. It certainly reveals the power of intent and demonstrates the significance of formulas from the last chapter:

- *Frequency + Intent = Healing*
- *Vocalization + Visualization = Manifestation*
- *Sound + Belief = Outcome*

This doesn't mean that there aren't individual frequencies for treating specific conditions, but simply that there's no single "magic" frequency that will work for everyone. This may be what's so wonderful about the arena of sound healing: There are many different approaches, methodologies, and frequencies for treating different imbalances. What a gift!

••• Exercise 3 •••

Our own unique vibrations color every aspect of our being. One of the easiest ways for us to honor our own uniqueness is simply to bring our focus to the music we like and the different ways we might use it.

Begin to compile a list of different types of music that you might use for various activities, such as eating, relaxing, exercising, meditation, reading, or whatever you can think of. Try playing these varieties of music during the different pursuits and note how effective they may be. As an experiment, try mixing them around to see what happens. Is there a particular musical composition that you use for jogging? Do you have a favorite type of music that you put on for relaxation? Experience what happens if you try the tunes that you use for relaxation when you're jogging. You'll probably find that you have very specific musical tastes for different activities, and what works for one may not work for another.

If it's appropriate, share your music list with others and get their responses—this will probably give you another indication of our uniqueness as vibratory beings. There are no right or wrong answers. This exercise will simply expand your awareness of the effects of music and bring you the realization that no one type— no specific sound—will affect each of us in the same way.

• • ● ● ● • •

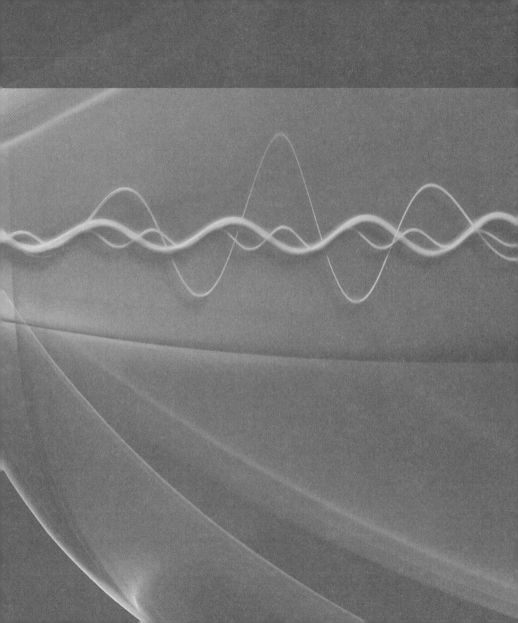

Secret 4

Silence
Is
Golden

It shouldn't be necessary to articulate this secret. It should be obvious to anyone reading this book. It should be obvious to anyone *writing* such a book . . . so how could I initially forget it? Why did it take a conversation with a colleague to make me remember it?

This secret wasn't even the main focus of the discussion that the two of us were having. We were talking about the changes in the sound-healing field over the last few decades: What was different? What had stayed the same? Why was it that many of the mentors I'd studied and trained with and

the colleagues and friends I'd taught alongside were no longer remembered? Why, as the field grew more popular and
mainstream, did it seem that some of the very fundamental
principles we'd discovered had been forgotten?

And in passing, my friend said something to effect of: "You
know, I can't believe that people don't realize that sound is a
subtle energy."

To which I responded: "Yes, I can't believe people think
that louder is better."

Our discussion then turned to the importance of silence
and how few people knew about its power. I happened to
have a notebook with me, and I snapped my fingers and wrote:
"Silence Is Golden." Thus, the title of this chapter, which hon-
ors the energy of silence, was created.

It's easy to see why this idea initially eluded me. Here in
the "supersize me" tradition of the West, our understanding is
often askew. We indeed believe that "bigger is better!" "louder
is better!" and "more is better!" And this includes our understanding of energy—and, in particular, subtle energy.

SUBTLE ENERGY

Sound is a subtle energy? *Yes!* What *is* subtle energy? . . .
Well, it's a bit difficult to define, but usually it's understood as

being any energy that can't properly or adequately be measured and understood by Western methods. This would include acupuncture, qigong, Reiki, Therapeutic Touch, electromagnetic therapy, light therapy . . . and, of course, our old friend sound healing. I used to joke that sound healing was the grossest form of subtle energy, because it was the *least* subtle, most physical, and perhaps most profound.

Sound travels as relatively slow, measurable waves, yet its uses and effects are the same as the subtler forms of energy—even that of light therapy. The only real difference is that we can feel the vibrations of sound more easily. Thus, while one aspect is quite measurable, there are other components—such as intent—which are quite difficult to validate, at least in current Western scientific terms.

A major key in understanding sound as subtle energy is the phenomenon of harmonics—the color of sound. Every sound that occurs in nature is actually a composite of multiple frequencies called *harmonics* or *overtones*. Just as white light is composed of all the colors of the spectrum, so the sounds that we hear—including musical notes on instruments or the tone of our voice—are in reality the multiple sounds of harmonics. Harmonics are responsible for the "timbre" or color tone of instruments and our voice—those that are most prominent and audible are responsible for the sounds created by different musical instruments, as well as the extraordinary variety of tonal quality that make each of our voices individual and unique. Our body, our brain, and in particular, our ears are extremely sensitive to the subtle effects of specific harmonics. Even though you may not be conscious of them, harmonics have been affecting you all your life.

Whenever a sound is created, such as that of a string being plucked, myriad other subtle tones—harmonics—simultaneously occur along with that first fundamental frequency of the string. These harmonics are multiples of the initial frequency, increasing by whole numbers. The second harmonic vibrates twice as fast as the first. The third harmonic vibrates three times as fast, the next vibrates four times as fast, and so on. All these sounds blend together, creating the tone color of the note. As they increase in their frequency, vibrating faster and faster (continuing conceptually into infinity), they become more and more subtle in nature. Thus, these harmonics contribute greatly to the subtle structure of sound.

Many people believe that much of the extraordinary healing power of sound is due to the harmonics. My first book, *Healing Sounds,* is in fact subtitled *The Power of Harmonics,* and it dealt with the phenomenon of harmonics in detail. The human voice has the remarkable ability to actually create distinct and audible harmonics, which make the tones projected even more powerful. Known as *vocal harmonics* or *overtone singing,* this ancient technique has been utilized in many sacred traditions, including Mongolian shamanism and Tibetan Buddhism. As we open more and more to the world of sound, the power and importance of harmonics becomes another aspect of vibration on which to focus our awareness and our intention.

As the field of sound healing continues to flourish and grow, many more people are discovering the power of sound to heal and transform; and as this becomes increasingly evident, many more people who lack experience begin to experiment with it. Thus, what's obvious and apparent to someone who has been in the field for a number of years may not be so to a neophyte who has just discovered the power of sound. At present, there are many books available about sound healing, but I don't recall seeing too many chapters with the *bigger is not better* concept. (*I've* never actually included it in anything that I've previously written.) Thus, I write this secret for all of us—for those who have yet to discover it and those who may have forgotten it.

THE IMPORTANCE OF SILENCE

Let's begin by acknowledging the power of silence. When I first got into sound healing, I didn't know about silence. I became so enamored with my own voice when teaching or doing a healing session that I never gave it much credence!

I'd go from one sound to another without honoring quiet. It took many years for me to realize the importance of the space between the sounds.

In reality, silence is the yin to sound's yang. It's the polar opposite of sound—and it's equally important. I now like to tell students that silence is really the place that gives sound the opportunity to create healing. It's the space where the transformational work of frequency shifting happens and change occurs—a powerful and sacred place that should be acknowledged and honored.

In my workshops, we'll sometimes chant a sacred mantra with a specific intention for an extended period of time—perhaps a half hour or more. This activity is extremely powerful, but it's during the time afterward when we sit in silence that the true transformational experiences occur. Occasionally it actually takes a few minutes after the chanting for the extraordinary rush of silence to envelop me and, at times, take me to transcendent places of spiritual ecstasy. It's as if the sound had anchored me to the earth, and once the chanting is over, my spirit can then fly on the silence.

In certain traditions the true path of sound is through silence. In surat shabd yoga, for example, adherents listen to and meditate on the inner sounds found in silence. Various internal tones, such as the rushing of water or the humming of bees, have been described by practitioners. An entire interior landscape of consciousness has been charted based on the inner sounds heard. Through this form of meditation, a practitioner is able to travel to different planes of consciousness on these internal sounds.

Silence and sound work hand in hand. From my perspective, neither is better than the other, but rather both need to be honored and utilized for healing and transformation. So often when we first discover the power of sound—particularly of our own vocalizations—we ignore or forget the importance of silence. We become enamored with tones and frequencies that can affect the world around us. However, it's also important to remember the power of silence as we progress into these realms of sound.

PROFESSOR GAVREAU

We must be aware that, indeed, "louder is not better." We need only recall the story of Joshua in the Old Testament and the destruction of the walls of Jericho to understand the power of sound.

More recently, in the 1950s, there were reports from France of a Professor Gavreau, an engineer who'd become interested in the effects of frequencies on the human body. Gavreau built a six-foot version of the whistle used by French police, which was powered by compressed air. Unfortunately, after Gavreau's lab assistants turned this giant whistle on, they died almost immediately from the rupturing of their internal organs due to the extremely high volume of sound—which could apparently also split concrete. The giant whistle and various other devices, as well as all blueprints and photographs of them, were confiscated by the French government and have yet to be released. As a footnote, I add, "Understandably so."

During one of his teachings in the U.S. in the 1980s, Dr. Peter Guy Manners showed slides of a French newspaper describing the misfortune, including a photograph of the giant penny whistle. As the inventor of the Cymatic Instrument, which uses the direct application of sound on the body for healing, Dr. Manners was only too aware of the power of sound and the need for control of it.

AMPLITUDE

Part of Secret 1, "Everything Is Vibration," involved an understanding of resonance. This is one way of measuring sound through its frequency—the number of waves per second—which defines the sound in terms of its rate.

There are other means of definition. In particular, one very important method measures its loudness or *amplitude*—the intensity of the sound or the amount of sonic energy inherent in it, which is measured in a unit called a *decibel* (db), named after Alexander Graham Bell. The following list shows some commonly heard sounds and their equivalent decibels:

- 120 db—Threshold of pain
- 115 db—Ship's engine room
- 110 db—Low-flying jet
- 105 db—Loud rock band
- 100 db—Riveting machine; subway train
- 95 db—Motorcycle
- 90 db—Noisy factory; loudest orchestra
- 85 db—Heavy traffic
- 80 db—Factory; average automobile
- 75 db—Vacuum cleaner
- 70 db—Normal conversation
- 60 db—Department store
- 50 db—Average office or living room
- 40 db—Quiet office; library
- 30 db—Quiet day in the country; softest orchestra
- 20 db—Whisper
- 10 db—Gentle breeze
- 0 db—Threshold of hearing

HEARING LOSS

In many countries, 85 decibels is considered to be the maximum permissible volume allowed for the duration of a working day. Continued exposure to sounds above this level, particularly those of 100 decibels or higher, can lead to hearing loss.

Sadly, we seem to be raising a generation (or perhaps *we're* even part of that generation) in which profound hearing loss has already occurred due to excessive volume levels coming from various sound sources. Such hearing loss is of great concern.

When you buy headphones for your iPod or whatever playback system you may be using, a warning about the dangers of excessive volume comes with the instructions. Many years ago, I was on a train and there was a young man with headphones listening to music several feet away from me. Despite the noise level of the moving train, I could clearly hear the song. I approached him and tapped him on the shoulder.

He looked up at me. "You know that loud sounds can make you deaf?" I shouted. He nodded and then turned away. Recently, I had a similar experience on an airplane with someone sitting several seats away from me who was using headphones.

As is the case in other aspects of life, we have many choices. Our hearing is precious and, if possible, we should attempt to preserve it as much as we can. Thankfully, the effects of exposure to loud sounds are commonly known. I trust, therefore, that it's not necessary to delve too deeply into this. However, to repeat what should be common knowledge: *Loud sounds are hazardous and ultimately will cause permanent hearing loss.*

Before moving on, though, I'd also like to consider another question that's less commonly asked: Can loud sounds also have other detrimental effects besides hearing loss?

SHATTERING A GLASS

As we discovered in the first chapter, a singer's voice can shatter glass if it matches the resonant frequency of that glass. However, shattering glass only occurs when too much amplitude, or sound intensity, is applied. Alfred Tomatis, M.D., a physician and pioneer in the field of sound, found that well-trained opera singers were capable of reaching 150 decibels inside their own heads when singing at full strength. This, incidentally, is loud enough for them to damage their own hearing.

Thus, using the glass as a metaphor for the body, if we apply this principle to the human body and take into account the story of Professor Gavreau and his giant whistle, we ought to be cautious about how much sound we project into an organ, for example. No doubt if these amplitudes could split concrete, Professor Gavreau was working with tremendous decibel levels. Therefore, it's probably good to err on the side of caution in this regard.

Many sound-healing and subtle-energy practitioners, in fact, feel that less is better—that the body and its associated fields actually respond more effectively to the application of gentle energy. Robert O. Becker, M.D., in his book *The Body Electric* (with Gary Selden), investigates the effects of electricity on the human body. He found that it was actually the more subtle electrical charges that have the greatest influence over the human cellular structure.

The same may be true with respect to sound. Few realize that in the East masters of energy-healing techniques such as qigong were often also trained martial artists. There are stories of these masters being able to immobilize an opponent from across the room with a loud sound. This, however, isn't the same level of intensity that these masters would use for healing, where the volume would be much less . . . and, of course, their intention would be very different.

SOUND AND PREGNANCY

I stress the importance of being aware of the volume of sound because at times I've seen things that have deeply disturbed me. I've observed people delivering tremendous amounts of sound energy to a person for the purpose of healing—sometimes with less-than-beneficial results.

In particular, I'm cautious about the application of sound to pregnant women. Few realize that the fetus is extremely sensitive to sound—this tiny, fragile being begins to respond to it somewhere between the 9th and the 12th week of gestation. I've sung gentle lullabies to the expanded belly of a expectant mother and even to a woman who was about to give birth. In fact, I've even created a recording to assist in the birthing process . . . but that's different from directly standing over a prone pregnant lady and blasting loud sounds into her belly with some sort of sound-creating instrument. In many shamanic traditions, no healing work is performed below the heart area in order not to adversely affect the unborn. This is due to the delicate nature of the fetus and the desire of the shaman not to inadvertently injure it.

I share this information with you and ask those who do use sound for healing to be conscientious about only applying the most gentle and soft tones when working with someone who's pregnant or with very young infants.

MY VERY LOUD VOICE

I have a very loud voice (I stress the word *very*) but most frequently when I utilize it for any sort of therapeutic or trans-formational outcome, I do so in a gentle and focused way. In addition, I'll use different instruments (from tuning forks to Cymatherapy Instruments), making sure that they aren't too loud.

Sometimes when people are new to the power of sound, they aren't sensitive to or aware of that power or aren't yet able to appreciate its subtlety. In fact, sometimes they simply can't pick up on the sound—at least not if it's gentle and quiet. This doesn't mean that it isn't working or isn't affecting them. *It is.*

For many, the ability to feel the vibrations of sound makes this one of the more appealing of the subtle-energy therapies, but due to inexperience and lack of understanding, misuse may occur. What tends to happen is that people really want to hear it and therefore need it to be LOUD in order to do so—*ergo,* louder is better. I suggest that such individuals begin to work with the power of silence in order to appreciate the more subtle aspects of sound. Balance is the key to healing.

A BALANCED RELATIONSHIP

Please note that in the formula *Frequency + Intent = Healing*, there are two components that are important for the outcome of any situation:

1. One I call the "frequency," but I use this as a metaphor for all aspects of the physical sound—including not only the cycles per second, but also the decibel level.

2. The other ingredient of this formula, "intent," is the consciousness behind the sound.

Both of these ingredients are important in order to generate healing. Students sometimes misinterpret this formula, assuming that it means that the intent of the sound is more important than the sound itself. This isn't the case—it's both the frequency *and* the intent: a 50/50 partnership between sound and consciousness, in an equal and balanced relationship to each other.

We always need to become aware of the physical effects of sound and honor this. For example, if it were my intention to calm someone down, I wouldn't shout in the person's ear, as the physiological response to the loud noise would create the opposite of the soothing effect I desired, regardless of my intent.

OTHER EFFECTS OF LOUD SOUND

Besides having the ability to cause hearing loss, loud sounds can also affect your nervous system, triggering the "fight or flight" response. Such sounds raise your heart and respiration rates and brain-wave frequency, causing the release of adrenaline and disruption of your immunological system. The next time you're startled by a loud noise such as a car horn or siren, check yourself out and note what you're experiencing physiologically. It's doubtful that such sounds will have done anything but disturb you; however, it's important to be aware of their effects.

I was once in Venice Beach, California, where many street performers put on shows. One such performer offered a $100 bill to anyone who could stand still while wearing a blindfold. He promised that he wouldn't touch the person in any way. All he or she had to do was stand still.

A young man, no doubt with plenty of testosterone (a hormone related to masculine aggression), stepped forward and flexed his muscles. He'd take the bet—there was no way that he was going to move. He was blindfolded, and for a few seconds he stood brave and stoic. Then the person who'd made the $100 offer quietly blew up a balloon, came up from behind, and popped it next to the blindfolded man's ear. That was all it took: The young man jumped a couple of feet, the audience laughed, and for me the power of loud sound was once again demonstrated.

Some years ago, several studies were conducted of two demographic populations that were very similar, except that one lived in a pastoral setting while the other resided in a noisy environment near an airport. The incidence of stress-related illness—heart attacks, cancer, and the like—was nearly 60 percent higher in the population that was constantly exposed to loud sounds.

The next time you're outside and hear a loud sound such as a lawn mower, pay attention to the way your body responds. Odds are, your heart will be beating faster, your breathing will be quicker and shallower, and you'll be feeling tense. I personally have little doubt that this "noise pollution," which is rampant in our society today, may be one of the leading factors contributing to stress and related illnesses.

When you're working with sound, either as a transmitter or a recipient, it's important to remember that bigger is not better—that louder isn't necessarily more healing. In fact, it can be the opposite.

••• Exercise 4 •••

The power of silence is extraordinary, but it's something that few of us take the time and the energy to experience. In certain systems of yoga, meditating on silence is considered to be the easiest and most powerful path to enlightenment.

This next exercise is relatively simple, yet it's probably one that you haven't tried—at least not since you were a child. It's designed to reintroduce you to silence and the power inherent in it.

Find a quiet environment where you won't be disturbed, and settle into a comfortable position. If you like, before beginning, repeat the very first exercise in this book (which focuses on listening to your external space), as it provides an excellent contrast to this one.

The first step in experiencing the power of silence is quite easy: Simply block your ears. Most people use their fingers to do so—usually the index finger of each hand—but some prefer to hold their palms over their ears. The purpose of covering your ears is to cut down external noise as much as possible so that you can begin to tune in to your internal sounds.

Now close your eyes. With your ears blocked and your eyes shut, begin to listen. As you tune in, you'll find an internal symphony occurring that you were probably unaware of. You'll become conscious not only of your heartbeat and your breath, but after a little while you'll probably be able to hear the blood pumping through your body. You may be aware of very high-pitched sounds as well as very deep ones, all of which are part of your bodily orchestra.

Listening in this manner is an extraordinary tool for appreciating the power of silence and of the inner sounds that accompany it. Some people find this exercise particularly effective as a meditation technique. There are even advanced spiritual disciplines that instruct practitioners to use these inner sounds to travel to other planes of consciousness!

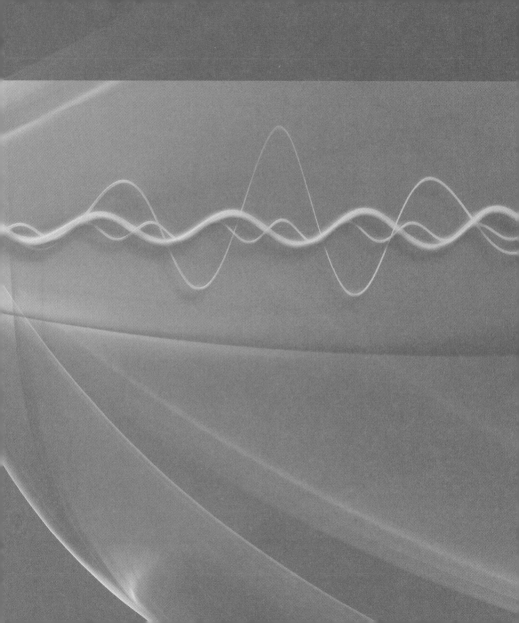

Secret 5

Our Voice
Is the Most
Healing
Instrument

This secret may be one of the most important that I share with you. It's simple and obvious . . . yet many of us have forgotten it or are unaware of its powerful nature. Therefore, to reawaken it in you, I now present this fifth and most valuable secret: *Our voice is the most healing instrument.*

Why the voice?

1. To begin, it's the most natural way to project healing sounds.

2. Second, it doesn't require batteries or electricity, so if you're in the middle of nowhere and need healing, you can just start making sound with your voice.

3. Third, an owner's manual isn't necessary. You don't have to go through special training or spend hours poring over pages and pages of material in order to learn to use it. You simply start making sound. In fact, you've been doing sound healing with your voice all your life.

Don't believe me? Just think back to a time when you may have hurt yourself. What did you do? You made a sound, I'm sure. Maybe it was "Ahh," "Oww," or whatnot, but it *was* a sound. You did it naturally, without thinking about it. And it probably helped ease the pain—in fact, I can almost guarantee that it did. If you want to prove this to yourself, the next time you stub your toe, try not to make a sound and see what happens. One thing I know is that it will hurt more! Anyone who has ever witnessed great physical or emotional trauma has heard all the groaning and moaning that accompanies these tragedies. People are expressing their pain through sound—the sound *lessens* the pain.

TONING

The use of the voice for healing is called *toning,* and it's probably the oldest and most natural form of sound healing that there is. Toning is often defined as using the voice to release pain; in addition, it's invoked to resonate different parts of the body, bringing them back into harmony and alignment.

Toning is the sounding of elongated vowels (such as *Ah*) or single-syllable sounds (such as *Om*). It's not the same as reciting sacred prayers or extended mantras such as Gregorian chants, Hindu kirtans, or Tibetan pujas, although, of course, all of these sound practices are powerful uses of the voice for healing and transformation.

Through toning, you can learn to find the frequency that works the best to resonate with you. Once you begin to use your voice in this manner, learning to experience vibrations with your own sounds, you can actually feel your utterances specifically resonate with different parts of your body. It's amazing—quite natural and very easy.

That's the first reason why your voice is the most healing instrument. Another is that your voice is the simplest and most effective way for you to project intention. It's much easier to put intent onto a sound you're making yourself than to project it onto a machine or instrument that you may be holding and be applying to someone else.

The next time you get a bellyache, try forming an "Oh" sound and gently focusing your attention on the part of your stomach that hurts while projecting the tone down there—this is often very helpful. The more you practice making sounds resonate with different parts of your body, the easier it will be.

Currently, there's limited scientific explanation for why toning is so effective, primarily due to lack of research. It has been suggested, however, that our own self-created sounds are an excellent way of helping our bodies release various chemicals and hormones, including dopamine, oxytocin, serotonin, and endorphins. Many of these neurochemicals relieve pain and may even make us feel ecstatic.

In his book *Self-Healing: Powerful Techniques,* Ranjie Singh, Ph.D., presents excellent research showing that certain sounds trigger the release of melatonin, a hormone that has been found to regulate the body's circadian rhythms and enhance sleep. It may even play a role in shrinking tumors. Other scientists believe that our tones can stimulate or relax the nervous system. Still others contend that toning can vibrate our entire being, oxygenating the body and brain.

A less-validated, although equally important, explanation for the effectiveness of toning is that individuals can learn to localize the specific resonance of their tones in different parts of their bodies. Using the principle of resonance, this can cause that which was vibrating out of harmony to come back into alignment.

I've personally heard testimonials from those who were able to effectively treat chronic conditions such as headaches and asthma through daily toning. I've also heard more remarkable anecdotal stories from people who claim they've been able to shrink tumors or heal broken bones in this way.

In her book *Sounding the Inner Landscape,* my friend and colleague Kay Gardner related how after breaking her toe in the middle of the woods, she was able to heal it on the spot through toning and then walk home. Such stories about the healing power of the voice are quite common.

If, as we've discovered, sound can change molecular structure, then by learning how to project different frequencies to specific parts of our body, we have the potential to heal any imbalance we may have. I've seen extraordinary healings occur through toning—and when they do, it does seem miraculous. (And, as I've previously mentioned, I've also seen *nothing* happen.)

ENTRAINMENT VS. ENTERTAINMENT

Many people inquire, "How can I use my voice for healing when I can't carry a tune in a bucket?" Another frequently asked question is: "If the voice is such a powerful healing instrument, why is it that so few people know about it?"

In Chapter 1, I referred to the phenomena of resonance and entrainment, which demonstrate the ability of one sound to shift the frequency of another. This is what happens when a part of the body begins to vibrate out of its normal, healthy resonance—it's the metaphor of the string player losing his or her sheet music and then having it returned. We can use sound to change the vibrations of a part of our physical or etheric body that may be weakened and out of tune and return it to a state of health. Our voice is the most accessible instrument to accomplish this.

You can hum a note or sound a tone that's not particularly musical—in fact, it may not even be pleasant for another person to hear. Yet if that sound is coupled with healing intention, it can be extraordinarily powerful. Here again is another example of the phenomenon of *Frequency + Intent = Healing*— using sound to change vibrational rates, which we refer to as *entrainment.*

Entrainment is not entertainment. If you get up in front of an audience and sing a song, that's most often entertainment— it's performance art. There's nothing wrong with this, but such an activity is usually not an example of sound healing. Most of the time amusing others in this way is very different from using our own self-created tones to resonate specific portions of our bodies. It's important that we differentiate between the two so that we realize that we can all learn to use the voice for healing and know that we don't need to be professional singers. When we resonate specific parts, these tones may not necessarily be pleasing—particularly to someone else—but they can be very powerful healing sounds.

Unfortunately, most people are still not aware of the healing power of their own voice. We've forgotten this remarkable natural ability. We've become confused about the power of our own self-created sounds, and instead of using them for our health and well-being, we've given this power of sound to others. We've created gods and goddesses who make sounds for us—we call them entertainers, divas, or even superstars. We worship them, buying not only their recordings, but following their adventures in magazines or on television shows. This is fine—it's great to honor skilled musicians and singers, but not at the expense of ignoring the healing power of our own voice.

Let's take back the power of our own sounds. We need to acknowledge and understand that we all have the ability to use our own self-created sounds to heal and transform. At the beginning of this chapter, I mentioned that this secret was both simple and obvious . . . and yet forgotten. Each of us has a voice, and we can use it—through toning—to help create health and balance for ourselves. Some who do so may find themselves led to other forms of making sound such as chanting sacred words of power. The only caveat is that you honor yourself and remember the other secrets of sound healing—in particular, that louder is not better.

When you make sound, be sure that it's comfortable and you don't strain or hurt your voice in any manner. Remember, also, that we're all unique vibratory beings and that entrainment isn't entertainment. Other than that, just enjoy yourself—through toning, an entire new world of transformation awaits you!

THE CHAKRAS

One of the most profound experiences that you can have with your own voice is through the resonance of your chakras. The word *chakra* is a Sanskrit term meaning "wheel." Perceived as spinning discs of light by those with the ability to see subtle energy, they are found in many traditions, including Hinduism and Tibetan Buddhism.

There are seven main chakras, located centrally in the front and back of the body. While they've been incorporated into many spiritual practices, the chakras seem to be based not on religion, but on awareness of energy. Scientific instruments are even beginning to record and validate their existence, as in the research of Valerie Hunt, M.D., described in her book *Infinite Mind.*

The next section of this chapter is devoted to the chakras, and in particular, to learning to use the voice to resonate them.

The purpose for this is quite simple: In doing so, we can balance and align them and thereby enhance our own self-healing by keeping ourselves in vibrational harmony. This can be considered a form of preventive medicine, and it's very effective. In addition, if a portion of the body (physical, emotional, mental, or spiritual) gets out of alignment, we can often put it back into balance simply through toning the chakras.

In this section, we'll begin to apply the secrets we've learned in order to create a practical and powerful method of sound healing that we can experience and use for ourselves.

The chakras are *transducers*—places where subtle energy from higher vibrational planes begins to become denser, until it's solidified as the physical body. Frequently, healers who work with subtle energy can detect imbalances before they manifest in the physical body by feeling them in the chakras. Therefore, by balancing the chakras, imbalances in the physical body often won't surface.

VOWELS AS MANTRAS

In workshops, I teach a number of different systems allowing participants to create sounds that will resonate with their chakras. One that I believe is particularly important is an exercise I developed called "Vowels as Mantras," which I've taught to many thousands of people throughout the world. In my workshops, I share a system of teaching that uses the sacred-vowel sounds in conjunction with pitch (another word for *frequency*). Those in attendance chant a specific vowel sound for each chakra in order to experience resonance there. This system is extremely powerful, and it's one that you'll have the opportunity to experience shortly.

When offered the opportunity to share a single special sound technique with an audience, I inevitably choose "Vowels as Mantras." My reasons for this are twofold.

First, whenever people do this exercise, they experience some form of resonance within their body, mind, or spirit. For many, it's one of the most extraordinary healing meditations they've ever done. There are those who find that being able to feel their voice resonating in different parts of their body is a life-changing experience.

The second reason for my enthusiasm for "Vowels as Mantras" as an exercise is this: The vowel sounds are sacred in many different traditions. This is something that very few people realize. Along with being profoundly powerful and revered tools of resonance, these sounds are nondenominational. No one has difficulty resonating with vowel sounds due to any prior belief system that might keep them from having this experience, as they're found in every language and therefore every culture and tradition. Thus, "Vowels as Mantras" is an ideal exercise for anyone who wants to discover the power of sound.

When doing this exercise in a workshop, I don't use a specified system of notes, pitches, or frequencies. Instead, I close my eyes, make a sound, and feel the part of my body associated with the corresponding chakra, as well as the energy center itself, resonate with it. This is how I can tell if the one I'm creating is correct for me or not; and if it's not, then I can adjust it. I usually start with the deepest note I can create in order to activate my root chakra and continue raising my pitch for the different energy centers. Most often I find that the highest sound I'm capable of making resonates with my crown chakra.

When I teach this exercise in a workshop, I use myself as the "conductor" for this chakra choir. After years of experience sounding my chakras, I'm able to find my specific resonance using my own voice. When I lead people in this exercise, I ask them to match my pitch. It works very well in large groups—I like to think of myself as some sort of tuning fork projecting a frequency that everyone can generically resonate with. Through this resonance—and our intention—the exercise is both healing and transformational.

However, after participants have experienced this in my workshop, I always suggest to them that the resonance of their own chakras won't necessarily match mine. When they experience "Vowels as Mantras" in the privacy of their own homes, they often find their own resonance to be unique. Frequently, when done alone, "Vowels as Mantras" is even more effective and powerful for them. (This exercise for toning your chakras with vowel sounds is presented at the end of the chapter.)

DIFFERING FACTORS

What's interesting about this particular system is that the actual resonance for my chakras seems to vary from day to day—the same note doesn't work every time. For example, the deepest one I'm able to sound changes, as does the highest.

In addition to teaching thousands of people "Vowels as Mantras" in workshops, I've developed the Healing Sounds Correspondence Course, an at-home study program that teaches them the technique I've been describing. Many students have gone through this 16-week course and reported back about their experiences. What I've discovered is that, like myself, participants have found that the sounds for their chakras do indeed vary from day to day, depending upon many different factors such as diet, sleep, exercise, and meditation. It seems that the resonance of our chakras can modulate and change in response to various physical, emotional, and mental activities.

• ● •

The exercise that you're about to embark on is "Vowels as Mantras." Before you begin, know that it can take up to a half hour to fully experience it, and I ask you to allow yourself adequate time for it. I'd also like to remind you to remain in your zone of vocal comfort as you make the sounds, not straining or experiencing any pain. Finally, I'm asking you to be aware of the importance of your intention as you make the sounds.

Remember to bring your awareness to each of your chakras and the part of the body where it's located while intoning these vowel sounds—it will make all the difference in your experience. The following illustration may prove helpful.

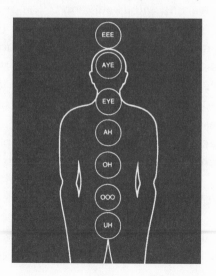

••• **Exercise 5** •••

Find a place where you can make sound and not be disturbed. Sit comfortably in a chair with your back straight, and stay as relaxed as possible. This exercise is often best experienced with your eyes closed.

— **1st Chakra:** Begin with the first chakra, called the "root" or "base" chakra, located at the base of the spine. Involved with the physical process of elimination and the organs that work with that function, it's the chakra associated with the energy of survival and with grounding to the physical plane.

The vowel sound for this chakra is the very deepest **"UH"** that you can make (as in the word *huh*). It ought to be soft and gentle, as should all the sounds you'll be making throughout this exercise. Focus your attention on the lowest part of your body and project your intention for the sound to resonate at the base of your spine. Feel it vibrating that area, and as it does, become aware that the energy center associated with this region is also resonating and becoming balanced and aligned through your sounds. Make this **"UH"** sound seven times (if possible).

— **2nd Chakra:** Focus your attention on the second chakra, called the "sacral" chakra, located about two to three inches below the navel. It's associated with sexual energy, the reproductive organs, desire, and creativity.

The vowel sound for this chakra is **"OOO"** (as in the word *you*). Begin to intone an **"OOO"** sound, making it a little less deep and slightly higher in pitch than the last one. Focus your attention on the area of the second chakra and project the sound into it. As it resonates the second chakra, experience this energy center balancing and aligning with the first chakra. Make this **"OOO"** sound seven times.

— **3RD CHAKRA:** The third chakra, often called the "belly" or "solar plexus" chakra, is located at the navel and a little above. Its energy is associated with digestion and the digestive organs, along with power and mastery of self.

The vowel sound for this chakra is **"OH"** (as in the word *go*). Begin to intone a very gentle and soft **"OH"** sound, which should fall within the midrange of your voice and be slightly higher in pitch than the last chakra. Focus your attention on your navel and project the sound to this area. As it resonates there, experience this energy center balancing and aligning with the other chakras. Make this **"OH"** sound seven times.

— **4TH CHAKRA:** The fourth chakra, often called the "heart" chakra, is located in the middle of the chest. On the physical level, it works with the lungs and the heart. Emotionally and spiritually, it's associated with the energy of compassion and love.

The vowel sound for this chakra is **"AH"** (as in the word *ma*). **"AH"** is often a sound we make when we're in love, and, indeed, the heart chakra is the center associated with this emotion. Begin to intone a soft and gentle midrange **"AH"** sound, higher in pitch than the last one. Focus your attention on your heart chakra and project the sound there. As you resonate your chakra with sound, experience this energy center now being balanced and aligned with the other chakras. Make this **"AH"** sound seven times.

— **5TH CHAKRA:** The fifth chakra, called the "throat" chakra, is located in the throat area. It's the energy center associated with the process of communication, speech, and hearing, as well as the ears and vocal apparatus.

The vowel sound for this chakra is **"EYE"** (as in the word *my*). Begin to intone a soft and gentle **"EYE"** sound, which is still higher in pitch than the last chakra. Focus your attention on the throat chakra and project sound there. As you do so, experience this energy center balancing and aligning with the other chakras. Make this **"EYE"** sound seven times.

— **6TH CHAKRA:** The sixth chakra, called the "brow" or "third eye" chakra, is located in the forehead between the eyes and slightly above them. It corresponds with imagination, psychic abilities, and opening to spiritual awareness. Mental activity and brain functions are also associated with it.

The vowel sound for this chakra is **"AYE"** (as in the word *may*—rather than the affirmative *aye*). Begin to intone a soft and gentle **"AYE"** sound, higher in pitch than the last chakra. Focus your attention on it and project the sound to the forehead area. As it resonates in the third eye, experience this energy center aligning and balancing with your other chakras. Make this **"AYE"** sound seven times.

— 7TH CHAKRA: The seventh chakra, called the "crown" chakra, is located at the top of the head. It's associated with complete resonance of spiritual energy. Said to control every aspect of the body and mind, it's normally not fully open in most humans. Pictures of saints and other spiritual beings with halos are indications of an activated crown chakra, wherein the individual becomes the embodiment of full enlightenment and union with God.

The vowel sound for this chakra is the very highest **"EEE"** that you can make (as in the word *me*). Begin to intone a soft and gentle **"EEE."** (For men, it may be helpful to use a falsetto voice to achieve this.) Focus your attention on your crown center and project sound to this area. As it resonates the crown chakra, experience this energy center being balanced and aligned with the other chakras. Make this **"EEE"** sound seven times.

Now remain momentarily in silence. For many, this period of quiet is the time to experience deep meditation. Enjoy it! When it's appropriate, open your eyes and spend a few minutes in profound appreciation of the experience you've just had.

· · ● ● ● · ·

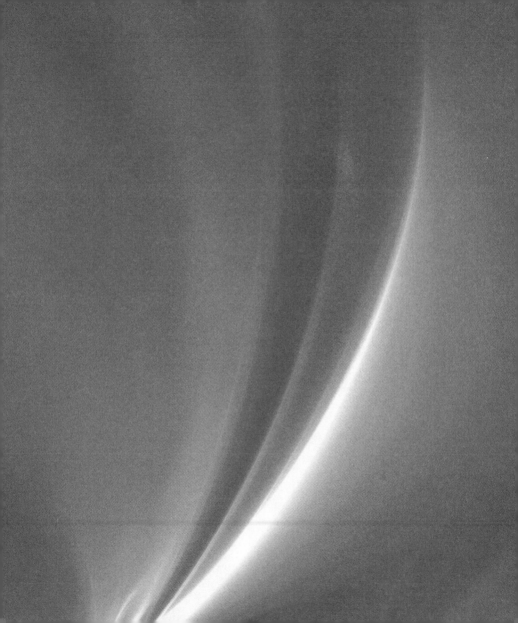

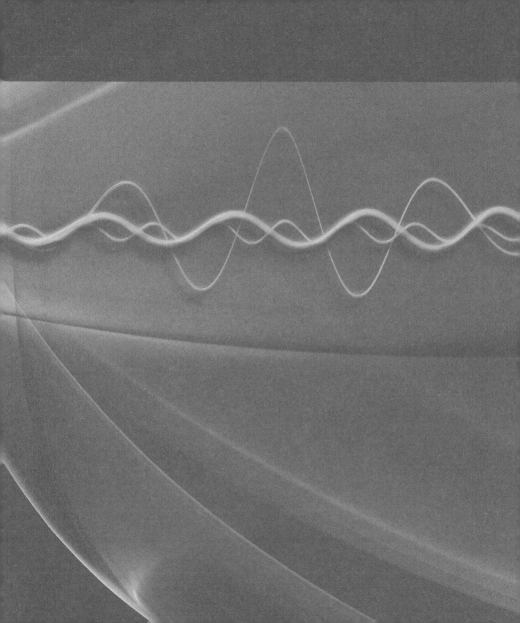

Secret 6

There Are
Many Notes
in a
Scale

The field of sound healing is vast. It encompasses so many different modalities—from using music for stress reduction to projecting vibrations into the body for frequency shifting. Sound healing is actually much like sound itself: There are many different types. If someone were to try to characterize a "sound," what would it be? A voice? An instrument? Thunder? A radio? The possibilities are endless.

In Western music, in order to delineate the different potential sounds that a musical instrument can create, the octave (the distance between one frequency and another, vibrating at twice the rate of the first) has been subdivided into 12 different and unique segments to form what's called a scale. The notes that comprise the scale are: C, C♯, D, D♯, E, F, F♯, G, G♯, A, A♯, and B. This is about as basic a division of music as can be made; indeed, each of these notes does have a different sound, feeling, and effect.

In addition, it turns out that there are many methods for dividing an octave, such that even those particular notes with the same name may vary in frequency among one other. This depends upon the particular tuning system that's used to divide them. In the United States, the note A on a piano has been assigned the frequency of 440 Hz. Most people therefore assume that it's always 440 Hz, but this isn't necessarily true. The note of A can resonate anywhere from approximately 432 Hz up to 448 Hz, for example, depending upon the part of the world and which system of tuning is used to create the scale. Any frequency from 432 Hz to 448 Hz can be defined as an A note. Thus, we have all sorts of variance with regard to what the different frequencies of specific notes actually are.

What started out as simply 12 notes has now manifested as hundreds, perhaps even thousands, of them, depending upon the system of division that's used. All of these are true notes— they may sound different and some may be more pleasing than others, but they're all real. And just as there are many different notes in a scale, so too are there many different approaches to sound healing. There are numerous diverse methods by which people project sound onto the physical self, the brain, the etheric fields, and subtle bodies in order to positively affect and change the body, mind, and/or spirit.

At this point, it's my intention to present some of the major modalities of sound healing that may be considered the basis of all other systems. Over the past 25 years, I've encountered many different types of sound healing, but for the most part, they all seem to fit into one of these categories. There are obviously methods, treatments, and the like that I haven't heard of—some may be very new; some may be very old, but they'll probably all adhere to the previous secrets revealed in this book, as well as fitting into one of these categories. In addition, some of the therapies that are currently being developed may combine two or more categories. Still, a basic understanding of each will be useful for readers interested in exploring sound healing.

Mantra Chanting

Undoubtedly one of the oldest uses of sound as a therapeutic and transformational tool (perhaps dating back thousands of years), mantra chanting is based on the concept that everything in the universe is in a state of vibration, and there are specific words or phrases that can manifest this vibration. Rather than using resonant-*frequency* healing, this therapy employs resonant-*word* healing. Thus, a client will sound specific mantras designed to create balance and alignment on the physical, emotional, mental, or spiritual level.

Mantras are sacred sounds of power, usually either single words or sentences from the Hindu or Tibetan tradition, although they can be found in many other traditions throughout the world. Depending on the mantra, the particular sound can have the ability to cure specific conditions, balance the chakras, or induce different states of consciousness.

Conditions that may be treated: all are potentially treatable

Benefits that may be received: improved health and heightened consciousness

TONING

Along with mantra chanting, this form of sound healing is unquestionably the oldest on the planet. As noted in Chapter 5, toning is the use of self-created sounds (most often elongated vowels) to resonate the physical, emotional, mental, or spiritual body. There are techniques in which practitioners can sonically scan clients and then project the apparently needed frequency into them. It's also possible for individuals to practice and experience these sounds themselves, vibrating different parts of their physical or etheric bodies.

Toning seems to employ the concept of resonant-frequency healing, with the practitioner using the sound to scan the body for imbalances. The proper frequency is then directed at the area that needs it, and healing occurs. Toning, like the chanting of mantras, appears to be among the most powerful practices when the ingredient of intent is added—which can be more difficult to do if a therapist is busy utilizing a complicated piece of instrumentation.

Toning is by far the most natural form of sound healing— we use it all the time, such as by moaning and groaning when we're in pain. It's also great for stress reduction. Anecdotal information exists about people with chronic (and sometimes terminal) conditions who have been healed through toning.

Conditions that may be treated: all are potentially treatable

Benefits that may be received: improved health and heightened consciousness

MUSIC THERAPY

Here in the West, music therapy is a very specific approach in which the practitioner works with clients, usually using songs and music, to help modify behavior. Often this is an interactive experience, with a music therapist playing songs for a client, and it frequently takes place in hospitals or institutions. As well as calming clients, music therapy has proven very effective for stress and pain reduction. It's also being initiated in hospice situations. There's an entire accredited music-therapy college-degree program, as well as certification through the Certification Board of Music Therapists.

Of the various modalities associated with sound healing, music therapy is one of the most accepted by traditional medicine. In many other parts of the world where allopathic treatment is less available, other forms of music therapy occur in which people sing songs, chant mantras, and do other sonic activities—with a high percentage of healings.

Conditions that may be treated: stress, pain, emotional imbalances, terminal illness/hospice

(**Note:** Nontraditional music therapy from around the world is used to treat any condition.)

Benefits that may be received: enhanced calmness, relaxation, pain reduction

RESONANT-FREQUENCY THERAPY

This therapy is based on the idea that every part of the body has a resonant frequency. Once an imbalance sets in, a cure can occur through restoring this resonant frequency. One of the first applications of this was Cymatic therapy (now called *Cymatherapy*), pioneered by Dr. Peter Guy Manners. The current machine offers more than 500 composite frequencies to treat different imbalances. What's most noteworthy about the Cymatic Instrument is that it uses a combination of five different frequencies, rather than a single tone.

Another very well-known machine on the market that uses a slightly different approach is the Rife instrument, invented by Canadian scientist Royal Rife. Rife was able to use a special microscope to view live viruses and bacteria and create different frequencies that would destroy them.

New machines based on the principles of these two instruments spring up all the time, with the aim either to enhance the resonant frequency of an organ (as in Cymatherapy) or use resonance to shatter an invading microorganism (similar to Rife therapy).

Conditions that may be treated: all are potentially treatable, from diseases of the physical body to imbalances of the chakras

Benefits that may be received: improved health—the Cymatic Instrument also transmits homeopathic remedies; the Rife instrument destroys various viruses, fungi, and bacteria

SONIC-ENTRAINMENT TECHNOLOGY

Pioneered by Robert Monroe and originally called Hemi-Sync, this technology uses a series of slightly out-of-sync frequencies to induce sonic entrainment. A client listens to binaural beat frequencies via headphones in order to balance the left and right hemispheres of the brain and help stimulate specific brain-wave activity.

Most of these sonic-entrainment techniques are focused more on enhancing consciousness than physically healing specific conditions, although heightened consciousness can also create physical improvement, as there's an interrelation-ship between the mind and body. Because the actual technology to create sonic entrainment is relatively simple, there are many such instruments and recordings that feature it. Among the most well known are the work of Robert Monroe, Kelly Howell, Joshua Leeds, Dr. Jeffrey Thompson, Anna Wise, and Tom Kenyon.

It's interesting to note that many indigenous cultures use sonic instruments that produce binaural beats, such as Tibetan bowls and Peruvian whistling vessels. Thus, Monroe's work may actually be many thousands of years old . . . ancient knowledge now rediscovered.

Conditions that may be treated: stress, emotional issues, learning disabilities

Benefits that may be received: relaxation, heightened consciousness, enhanced learning

AURAL-ENHANCEMENT TECHNOLOGY

This technology and the program that accompanies it—most often called the Electronic Ear—was developed by Alfred Tomatis, M.D., an otolaryngologist from France. Sometimes called the "Einstein of the Ear," Tomatis researched the interrelationship between the ear, hearing, and the body for more than 30 years. According to Tomatis, there are three functions of the ear: (1) to assume balance, (2) to allow us to hear, and (3) to charge the brain. This sense organ is also extremely important in the development of spatial awareness and language.

The Electronic Ear uses a series of specially filtered music (frequently Mozart or Gregorian chanting) that a client listens to via headphones. Tomatis found that the ear was responsible for providing much of the energy charge to the brain. He discovered that certain sounds fatigued the ear, brain, and body, while others were stimulating. Designed to open the ear and the brain up to greater sonic frequencies, the Electronic Ear and similar devices treat imbalances such as learning disabilities and dyslexia, as well as emotional issues.

Guy Berard, M.D., a colleague of Tomatis, developed his own program, called Auditory Integration Training (AIT), based on related research. While not as well known as Tomatis's Electronic Ear, Berard's work claims equal success in similar areas. In recent years, therapists such as Ron Minson, M.D., have combined the work of Tomatis with the sonic-entrainment technique of Robert Monroe to create intriguing and powerful treatments.

Conditions that may be treated: learning disabilities, dyslexia, exhaustion, impaired motor skills, problems with language development

Benefits that may be received: enhanced learning, improved language development, increased energy

VOICE-ANALYSIS THERAPY

This therapy, pioneered by Sharry Edwards, focuses on analyzing the voice, determining frequencies that are missing, and finally playing them back to create harmony and healing in the client. According to Edwards and others who approach sound from this perspective, the missing frequencies in the voice relate to imbalances in the emotional, mental, or physical body. Reintegrating them is the key to restoring clients' health.

Some suggest that these frequencies can be related to the atomic weight found in the periodic table of elements. Various practitioners who use this modality of sound therapy can at times be in agreement or at odds over the meaning of a frequency. Different sources of analyzing the voice also exist—from complicated digital instrumentation to tuners of acoustic instruments.

Vocal analysis reveals very specific frequency imbalances that may be occurring in an individual. The treatment usually incorporates playing back these sounds as single-tone frequencies. Some practitioners use synthesizers to do so; others actually employ samples of the human voice. Some of the better-known technologies using this approach are Edwards's own BioAcoustics, as well as Sound Wave Energy and BioWaves.

Conditions that may be treated: all are potentially treatable

Benefits that may be received: improved health

VIBROACOUSTIC THERAPY

This therapy uses specially designed tables, beds, and chairs in which a client will sit or lie down and receive specific frequencies or music that's generated through the sonic furniture and projected into the body. Such devices include the Somatron, the BETAR, and the Genesis Bio-Entrainment Module, among others. Some of these devices are simple yet effective, such as the So Chair, which implants the transduction of sound from CDs into the body. This is quite relaxing, powerful, and transformative.

Other vibroacoustic therapies utilize more sophisticated equipment, often combining several of the other techniques described in this chapter. For instance, the Genesis machine, created by Michael Bradford, includes a computer that's able to analyze aspects of the frequencies the body needs for healing and then generate those particular sounds. Tables and instruments, such as those used by Dr. Jeffrey Thompson at the Center for Neuroacoustic Research, project therapeutic frequencies utilizing the sound of the person's voice.

Conditions that may be treated: stress, muscular problems (depending upon the specific frequencies being projected, potentially any condition can be treated)

Benefits that may be received: relaxation, heightened consciousness, improved health

TUNING-FORK THERAPY

This modality of sound healing, pioneered by Dr. John Beaulieu, uses specially designed tuning forks for relaxation and balance. In particular, the most popular and effective method employs two aluminum tuning forks that are cut to specific frequencies or ratios. They're then sounded together and brought about three inches away from each ear. When applied in this manner, they seem to affect the ears, brain, and nervous system, bringing balance and alignment.

The most common and effective ratio for these tuning forks is 2:3—creating the musical interval of the perfect fifth, considered sacred in many traditions with an understanding of the relationship between mathematics and the cosmos. Legend tells that Pythagoras, the ancient Greek philosopher and musician, believed that the ratio of 2 to 3 was extremely therapeutic. Thus, these instruments are sometimes called *Pythagorean tuning forks.*

During the listening process, the physical body aligns with the interval created by the tuning forks, creating balance in the nervous system. These tuning forks also balance the left and right hemispheres of the brain, reducing brain-wave activity and inducing states of relaxation. Since tuning forks can be cut to any ratio or frequency, the sound-healing market is presently flooded with many different ones of varying ratios and frequencies whose marketers claim extraordinary results.

Conditions that may be treated: nervousness, headaches, exhaustion, energy imbalances

Benefits that may be received: stress reduction, relaxation, energy enhancement, balance of the nervous system and etheric fields

SONOPUNCTURE

Sonopuncture is the term for the projection of sound, rather than needles, into the acupuncture points and meridians of traditional Chinese medicine. While conceivably any kind of sound projector or applicator, such as a massage vibrator, can radiate sound into the body for this purpose, tuning forks have become the most common application of sonopuncture. In contrast to their use described in the preceding section—in which they don't touch the body and are used as tools for listening, affecting the brain and nervous system—with this approach, the stems of the tuning forks are applied to the body and actually come into contact with skin.

This method of healing uses the meridian system of traditional Chinese medicine. As with other therapeutic approaches, there are many different systems that can be utilized in this treatment. Some practitioners use the same single tuning fork for all the points and meridians. Others use two or more specifically tuned forks—one for each point or meridian. Among the many names for this form of sound therapy are BioSonics and Acutonics.

Conditions that may be treated: all that are treatable by acupuncture

Benefits that may be received: correction of any imbalances treatable through acupuncture

NATURAL ACOUSTIC INSTRUMENTS

One of the most flourishing sound-healing modalities involves the use of acoustic instruments, including crystal bowls, Tibetan bowls, Peruvian whistling vessels, and didgeridoos. Many of these are indigenous in origin—such as the wooden didgeridoo, which is from Australia; or bowls made of seven semiprecious metals, which come from Tibet or Nepal—and can be found in ancient traditions that understood the power of sound to heal and transform. These instruments are sounded near or on the body to create balance and harmony.

Among the most popular of these acoustic tools are quartz-crystal bowls, which seem to have only been in existence for the last 25 years. One of the reasons for their popularity is quite simple—anyone can take the little rubber mallet that comes with the bowl, rub it around the outside (just as you'd rub your finger around a wine glass to produce a tone), and generate a sound that's quite amazing.

The sound of these bowls is entrancing, and many people experience profound therapeutic and transformational effects simply by listening to them. Certain medical professionals use them for stress reduction and enhanced relaxation.

Conditions that may be treated: stress, energy depletion, chakra imbalance

Benefits that may be received: relaxation, energy enhancement, chakra balancing

COMPACT DISCS

No list of modalities would be complete without mention of CDs with specifically designed frequencies, either generically created for a general purpose such as relaxation, enhanced learning, or chakra balancing or specifically designed for the imbalance of a particular client. Often these CDs will simply be recordings of the sounds from the different modalities described in this chapter. With an experienced and knowledgeable creator, some will combine them (such as Monroe's Hemi-Sync and the technology of Tomatis's Electronic Ear, coupled with Pythagorean tuning forks and mantras from various traditions, along with other sound-healing knowledge) to create new, different, and powerful therapies.

No doubt many of the different CDs that are available are extremely useful and effective. Some of them may rely mainly on the placebo effect, in which no sounds of specific efficacy are actually present, but the belief in the listener is enough to create healing and transformation. Because of their inexpensiveness, CDs reporting to possess extraordinary healing abilities now flourish in the sound-healing market.

Conditions that may be treated: stress, learning disorders, exhaustion, pain (depending upon the CD and the sounds, potentially any condition can be treated)

Benefits that may be received: relaxation, sleep enhancement, pain reduction, improved learning, increased energy, chakra balancing, heightened consciousness

• ● •

These categories are by no means inclusive of all the various possibilities inherent in the field of sound healing, and are listed simply to give some examples of the potential treatments found in the field. In truth, the arena of sound healing is limitless—as I mentioned, it's like an extraordinary pie in which there are many different slices (or approaches) that are very different, yet all may be successfully applied and utilized for healing and transformation.

I always like to suggest that from my perspective, there's no therapeutic, educational, or transformational modality that can't be enhanced by using some aspect of sound, since it has the extraordinary ability to manifest change. What's most exciting is that despite all the amazing inroads that have recently occurred, sound healing is still in its infancy. The future of this field may bring us greater surprises than we can ever imagine!

••• Exercise 6 •••

There are many different forms that sound healing can take. Go over the list of modalities that have been presented in this chapter. Was there a specific form of sound healing that seemed most appealing to you? Perhaps you felt a certain resonance with one in particular. Remember your connection with this modality, and when the opportunity presents itself, allow yourself to experience it. You've already been exposed to the power of toning with the exercise in the last chapter.

Right now you can experience another one of the modalities that were described herein—that is, listening to CDs. *Peaceful Journey,* the recording that's been included with this book, was created to reduce stress and enhance relaxation. When you have about a half hour available, allow yourself the opportunity to experience this recording. (Incidentally, it's perfectly fine if you've already listened to it.)

1. For this exercise, first begin by taking a few minutes to observe yourself. How do you feel? Are you stressed or relaxed? What is your breathing like? How is your pulse rate?

2. Find a comfortable place where you won't be disturbed, take out the CD that accompanies this book, and listen to the recording of *Peaceful Journey.*

3. When the sound stops, observe yourself again: Do you notice any difference in how you now feel? Do you feel better or worse than before?

4. Please read the information about the CD at the end of the book. This recording features a number of different sounds, tones, and frequencies that are designed to put you into deep states of relaxation. Sometimes the process of education can enhance the effects of what you're experiencing—particularly when it comes to music.

5. Now listen to the recording of *Peaceful Journey* again, and see if reading the information makes any difference in your listening experience. If it does, that's excellent. If not—and you have a negative response—that simply means that this recording isn't right for you and you shouldn't listen to it again. Instead, please go on to the next chapter; thus, the CD just doesn't resonate with you.

Remember that there are many notes in a scale, and if *Peaceful Journey* didn't work for you, there are many other sounds that will!

* * ● * *

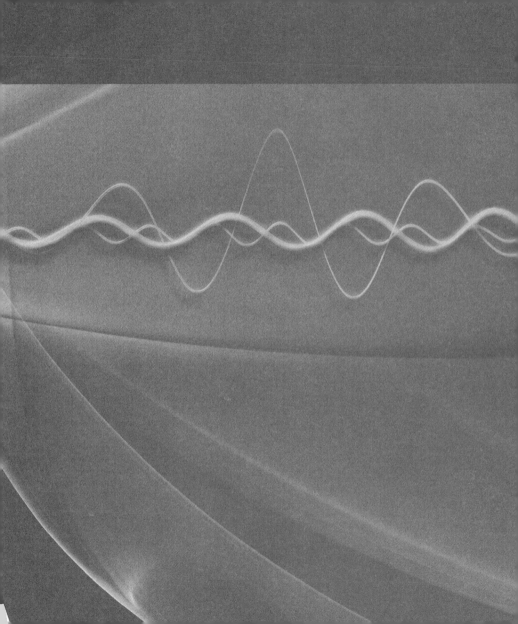

Secret 7

Sound Can Change the *World*

Until now, the primary focus of this book has been on the use of sound to create positive change on a personal level—that is, with ourselves or, if we're practitioners, with clients. However, there's another level where sound can be used to effect change: the level of the world itself.

I doubt anyone would argue that we live in tumultuous times. There are many books written on this subject alone. As we progress into the 21st century, there are planetwide issues at stake—issues that must be addressed: famine, disease, genocide, pollution, global warming, war . . . the list could go on and on. Many traditions perceive this as being a time of remarkable change and transition. Some call it the "End

Times" or "The Great Shift." Regardless of what name you give it, this particular juncture seems to be very special and merits our immediate attention.

Fortunately, most of the issues that need to be resolved are human made. Some, no doubt, are naturally occurring, but even a close examination of these seems to show humans as their basis. As such, these issues can be resolved through human intervention: We created it, so we can fix it.

The focus of consciousness and activity that's needed to fix these issues demands cohesive global unification. One person, even one country, can't make the changes necessary to repair all the damage that has been done through negligence, denial, and pure foolishness. All the beings on this planet must work together as one.

In certain indigenous cultures, it was said that no action would be taken until its ramifications had been considered down through seven generations. A tree wouldn't be cut down in order to provide warmth for a fire if doing so would damage the fragile ecosystem where it was growing. These cultures knew how to keep things in balance.

Today, whether it's the destruction of the rain forest, the spread of disease, or genocide, there's little balance. This needs to change.

The solution to the question of how to create this change isn't easy—the human race as a species needs to evolve to a level of consciousness where we understand that we can no longer exist as solitary units who remain isolated from one another. In other words, we must learn to work together as a compassionate and caring species, assisting each other, and as we do, assisting the planet itself. This learning to cooperate with each other needs to be taught. Through such education and awakening, we may achieve global consciousness.

The question, of course, is: *How do we do this?* One answer is: by working with "intentionalized" sound. We need to understand, honor, and utilize the power of sounds when they're created with consciousness.

Throughout this book, I've stressed that for personal healing to occur, the formula *Frequency + Intent = Healing* and its corollaries, *Vocalization + Visualization = Manifestation* and *Sound + Belief = Outcome,* are vitally important. Our intentions, visualizations, feelings, and beliefs are all able to amplify the power and effect of sound. Conversely, sound, frequencies, tones, and vocalizations are all able to boost the power and enhance the effects of our meditations and prayers. Together, these two elements of sound and the consciousness encoded within it combine in a synergistic manner to create a truly unstoppable force that can move mountains. It's no accident that most prayer on this planet is chanted aloud—the ancients knew of the ability of sacred sound to amplify and empower our prayers. We're once again beginning to rediscover this.

A number of different scientific studies have validated the effect of meditation and prayer on a planetary level, including the Global Consciousness Project at Princeton. Through the use of random-number generators (called EGGs) spread at points throughout the world, researchers have found that during certain events in which the consciousness of proportions of the population are engaged, the numbers from these EGGs become less random. When this occurs, the data may be collected and the numbers charted. Anyone who has ever seen the results of this knows that it creates a wave—which seems to indicate that global events are measurable. It's almost as though the consciousness of the planet can be charted through these EGGs.

In order to be registered via the EGGs, these global events aren't based on excitement, such as the Super Bowl. Instead, they must affect the shared emotions of the consciousness of those involved in them. In particular, the emotion of compassion seems to be of primary importance in this regard. Events of a cataclysmic nature, such as an earthquake or a tsunami, can be charted; so can positive ones such as global meditations and peace prayers.

Studies on Transcendental Meditation (TM) have also shown the positive effects of meditation and prayer on global events. As Gregg Braden notes, in studies such as that appearing in a paper published in *The Journal of Conflict Resolution,* there's data to indicate that during peace meditations violent behavior in the areas where they occurred declined considerably. The power of our consciousness is astonishing.

What perhaps is even more profound is that the number of people required to create a noticeable change in the consciousness of the planet is quite small. There's a critical mass necessary to manifest change—it's the square root of one percent of the population. On a planet of more than six billion people, this number is approximately 8,000 individuals. Only a mere 8,000! Think about that! In order to make a change in the consciousness of the planet, only a tiny percentage of people engaging in an activity or event such as a global meditation or peace prayer is necessary.

Many of you may be asking, "Well, if such a small number of people are required to create a shift and change this planet, then why don't we already have peace? There are certainly antiwar demonstrations with more than 8,000 people taking part!" This is quite true, but it's important for us to understand that while the numbers may be great at these demonstrations, the focused, coherent consciousness may not be.

In order to meditate and project the consciousness of peace, we must be in a peaceful frame of mind, feeling and focusing the energy of peace. Many who take part in these demonstrations no doubt ultimately desire peace, but they may also be quite angry, or they may be thinking about lunch, or they may be otherwise focusing their consciousness on something other than peace. The exercise at the conclusion of this chapter presents one method of projecting peace. While it's not difficult, as you'll observe, it is quite different than carrying a placard and shouting a slogan.

When I meditate, at times I receive guidance. I can't truly say who or where this guidance comes from, but when it occurs, it's usually correct and extremely important for me. More than 25 years ago, while deep in meditation, I became conscious that part of my purpose for being on this planet was to help introduce awareness of the healing nature of sound.

More recently, during a meditation, I asked for personal guidance with regard to my next step. After the quarter of a century I'd been engaged in this work, sound healing was now reaching mainstream proportions. I'd clearly helped carry out the purpose of introducing awareness of it. What, if anything, was next? I then received guidance that directed me to turn my own focus of awareness from personal-healing sounds to *planetary*-healing sounds. It was that simple—and that profound—for me.

I then began to investigate what it would take to create these planetary-healing sounds. Thankfully, it was nothing that I didn't already know. Still employing the variations of formulas on sound and consciousness that had become so vital to my teaching, I now realized that instead of projecting *Frequency + Intent* for another person's healing, we could simply project this energy for the planet.

Thus, for the past several years, my focus has not only been on using sound to heal us personally—on a physical, mental, emotional, and spiritual level—but also doing so to assist the planet. Beginning in 2003, I initiated World Sound Healing Day, which takes place every February 14—Valentine's Day. On this date, thousands of people throughout the planet intone the "Ah" sound, encoded with the intention of peace and harmony, sending a sonic valentine of love throughout the world. These planetary toning events also take place at other times throughout the year, and they do make a difference.

"Ah" for most people is simply a vowel sound and defies association with any spiritual denomination. Thus, it's acceptable for most people to make this sound, regardless of their background, culture, or religion. In reality, the "Ah" sound is one of the most powerful sounds on this planet, particularly useful for generating compassion. It's a sacred seed syllable and is considered to be a powerful mantra in many Eastern traditions, including Tibetan Buddhism. It's also a vowel sound—a divinely inspired tone considered sacred in many different traditions, including kabbalah. The "Ah" sound is found in most of the god and goddess names on the planet (Tara, Buddha, Krishna, Yahweh, Jehovah, Yeheshua, Allah, Saraswati, Wakan Tanka, Kuan-yin, and so on), as well as many sacred words (*amen, alleluia, aum*).

Most mystical traditions that work with the vowel sounds in relation to the chakras find that the "Ah" sound is associated with the heart chakra, the center of love and compassion. Thus, on World Sound Healing Day, people throughout the world generate an "Ah" sound, sending this energy of love and compassion across the planet.

Sound amplifies the intention. Although the "Ah" tone is recommended, any sound that people feel comfortable with is a good one, as long as they're feeling the energy of love and compassion when they make it. Sacred sounds aren't in competition with each other—in fact, they work together synergistically.

If you'd like to experience the power of sound firsthand, it's very easy. Simply find someone—perhaps a friend, partner, spouse, or offspring—and ask the person if he or she would be willing to take part in a sonic experiment. Once he or she has agreed to this, the next part is even easier: Explain that the next time you both find yourselves embroiled in some sort of disagreement, instead of going off in a huff (or worse yet, using the power of sound in a negative fashion by shouting profanities at each other), agree to make a gentle sound together.

Making this verbal contract ahead of time is very important so that in the heat of the moment, hopefully, one of you will remember your agreement and initiate sounding together. An "Ah" sound is highly recommended, as is an "Om." Or, as noted, use whatever you feel comfortable with, as long as it's a gentle and sacred sound.

What will almost invariably happen is that within a minute or two, the anger and whatever else you're feeling will be replaced by something much more positive. Chanting together allows you to attune to and resonate with each other. Your heartbeat, respiration, and brain waves will entrain with each other through breathing together and then sounding the "Ah." You both begin to create a field—one of kindness and compassion—and the end result is that it eases and often dissipates whatever discordant energy may have been about to manifest.

If you continue to make the "Ah" sound while focusing on the energy of love and appreciation, then that's what will manifest. As you make sound together, the barriers of separateness that create the illusion of duality—that we're not part of the sameness—disappear. It's extraordinarily powerful . . . and perhaps one of the key ingredients for creating planetary change.

As soon as you've experienced the power of sound to transform the energy of an argument on a personal level, it's time to become aware of the power of sound to shift the consciousness of the planet on a global level. If possible, join with others during any of the many global-peace events taking place. If they don't already know about the power of sound to amplify their consciousness and thoughts (and they may not), *let* them know.

Remember that in Dr. Emoto's water experiments, polluted and muddy-looking water became clear and crystalline after it had been prayed over. So our vocalized prayers have the ability to change not only molecular structure, but both personal and planetary consciousness as well.

Sound is a multidimensional energy, and it adheres to the constructs of modern quantum physics, which suggest that time and space don't really create the limitations that we believe they do. Experiments have shown that electrons separated by significant distances can be simultaneously influenced and affected by consciousness. So can our DNA. Our feelings, intentions, and beliefs seem to be major components of this. Sound is able to amplify these ingredients and thus enhance our ability to effect change in the very creation of reality.

As I've mentioned, Gregg Braden has written several important books on the power of prayer as well as the interconnection between all of us. It has been my great honor to have taught with Gregg—he truly understands the importance and power of both sound and belief.

A major insight that Gregg shares is that when the actual mechanism of a miracle is understood, it then becomes a technology. Our ability to encode our intent—our beliefs and feelings—upon a sound in order to manifest change can indeed create miracles. This ability may now be considered a technology . . . and this technology has the potential to change the world.

I encourage each and every person reading this book to utilize this profound technology of encoding sound with consciousness in order to make a difference. You don't need to wait for a global event in order to begin doing this—you can start right now.

One of the many ways you can do this is through the *Temple of Sacred Sound,* a new Internet Website that utilizes sound coupled with intention to assist global harmonization—enhancing harmony and peace on both a personal and planetary level. Our Website (**www.TempleofSacredSound.com**) is available for all to use 24/7, anytime of the day or night worldwide. Currently, the Internet represents the neural net of the earth—the Global Mind. Through sound, coupled with loving and compassionate intentions, we can activate the Global Heart of the planet and link body, mind, and spirit.

Temple of Sacred Sound has different sacred sound chambers where people across the globe can use the Internet to sound together with intention and resonate with each other. This sacred cyberspace sound temple can be used for special occasions such as World Sound Healing Day, as well as daily in order to enhance consciousness. Through Temple of Sacred Sound, the energies of sound, light, and love are generated in order to manifest peace and harmony for personal and planetary healing.

The next exercise is most helpful in order to assist you in the creation of planetary healing sounds. Read through the following steps and then try the exercise. You'll find that such an activity is mutually beneficial: Heal the planet and we heal ourselves; heal ourselves and we heal the planet!

••• Exercise 7 •••

Some of the most important feelings/intentions/consciousness that can be encoded upon a sound are those of kindness, compassion, appreciation, and love. These qualities truly seem to amplify not only the effect of the sound, but also the electromagnetic field that surrounds us. This is all measurable and verifiable.

1. First, find yourself a nice, quiet space where you won't be disturbed. Now, begin to think of something that you feel appreciation for— it could be a person; a pet; or even a scene that has brought you comfort, such as lying on the sand near the ocean. Feel the energy of appreciation in your heart as you continue to visualize whatever it is.

2. Now slowly begin to breathe in and out. As you inhale, feel the breath entering not only your nose and mouth, but also your heart. As you exhale, feel your breath moving out, not only through your nose and mouth, but also through your heart. Breathing in this manner is a powerful and important tool for enhancing deep relaxation and meditation. You're actually creating a coherent wave between your heart

and brain. You're also amplifying the electromagnetic field that's generated by both these organs.

3. Continue breathing in and out with this feeling of appreciation. Now, as you exhale, make a very gentle "Ah" sound filled with this energy of appreciation. Continue feeling the energy of compassion and unconditional love on this "Ah" sound.

4. When it feels appropriate, increase the volume of the "Ah" sound, but remember to keep it in your comfort zone. As you feel love and appreciation, kindness, and gratitude, know that this energy is being amplified and carried on the sound.

5. Some like to visualize the sound surrounding the planet and bathing Earth in this wonderful energy of peace and harmony. If you prefer, simply continue breathing, knowing that as you sound, you're resonating in a state of gratefulness, and that this energy is being transmitted to the world.

That's all it takes, and it *can* make a difference. You can change the world!

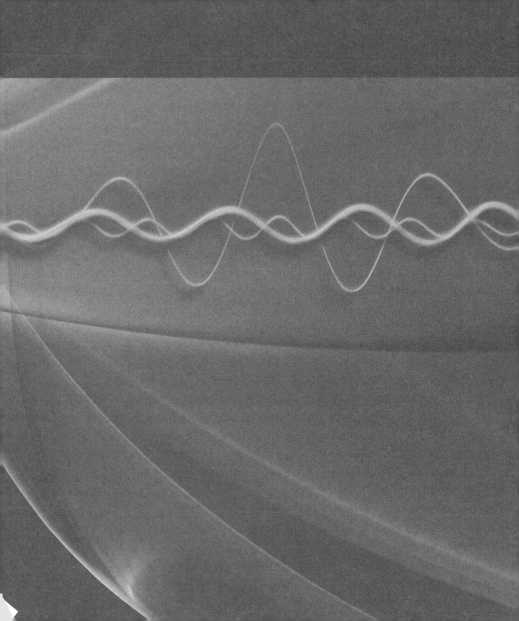

Afterword

In the Middle East, there was a man named Akbar, who had a beautiful instrument hand carved out of wood with many strings that could be plucked and sounded. Every day for hours on end, he played this instrument, striking the same string and the same note over and over. Finally, his wife could take it no more.

"Beloved husband," she began, "I must talk with you. You have this beautiful instrument with many remarkable strings that can play so many different notes and melodies. Your friends have the same instrument, and they use all these different strings, creating wondrous and varied sounds on it—different tunes and different songs. But you, beloved husband, sit here all day long, striking that same note over and over, again and again. Why do you do that? Why do you not play like your friends, creating many different sounds and melodies? Why do you keep hitting that same string over and over, again and again?"

Akbar smiled lovingly at his wife. "My dear wife," he said, "the reason my friends all play so many different strings and I do not is quite simple: They are still looking for their note, while I have found mine."

This brief story may be a metaphor for the information in this book. After all is said and done, it's important for each of us to find our note. Every frequency has a different energy. Each sound displays a particular essence. Combinations of frequencies and sounds create different and varied energies and essences. As I noted in the Preface, the field of sound healing is vast, and there are many different approaches and modalities to choose from. Find one and begin to explore it.

Let us briefly review the 7 Secrets:

1. Everything Is Vibration
2. Intent Is Powerful
3. We Are Unique Vibratory Beings
4. Silence Is Golden
5. Our Voice Is the Most Healing Instrument

6. There Are Many Notes in a Scale
7. Sound Can Change the World

Through understanding and utilizing these 7 Secrets, we can begin to experience the enormous power of sound to heal and transform. We can begin to resonate to different frequencies and to explore the vast network of sonic modalities that can be used to create positive change for ourselves and for others.

Akbar's story tells us that we must all find our own note. There's truth to that statement. Pythagoras, the ancient Greek father of geometry, philosophy, and music theory, was said to have declared that by observing and experiencing the sound of a single vibrating string, one could know the secrets of the universe. There's also truth in that. And there's truth in the fact that by experiencing many of the extraordinary sounds that exist throughout this planet, we can begin to taste the exquisite nectar that embodies the extraordinary spectrum of sound.

Thus, going from the alpha to the omega—from the beginning to the end—from fully experiencing one vibration to potentially experiencing as many as we can, we can still achieve the same result: that of finding our note. Using the secrets laid out is this book can make that task much easier.

Realize that sound is healing. Understand that everything is in a state of vibration. Acknowledge the power of feelings and intention to color the very universe we know. Accept that we're all unique vibratory beings and that there's no magic frequency—what works for one person may not work for another. Recognize that sound is a subtle energy and that bigger and louder aren't necessarily better. Know that our voice is the most healing instrument. Be aware that there are as many different notes in a scale as there are different approaches to using sound. Celebrate that we can change the world with our sound.

Despite the antiquity of sound healing, its development in our society is quite recent. We're still in the beginning stages with respect to accepting and understanding how sound can be used to heal and transform. And we don't know very much about sound itself. A lot of people may think that they do, but they're probably deceiving themselves. Sound is powerful. Sound is mystical. Sound is mysterious—it's extremely difficult to know anything except what works, or doesn't work, for you. And even this may change.

Nevertheless, using the secrets found in this book, you can have a solid grounding for coming to understand sound healing. Reflecting on these secrets will help develop your awareness of interfacing with sound as a tool for healing and transformation. Ultimately, you must see what works for you—what you feel comfortable with, what's most effective for you—that is, what resonates most deeply with you.

The world of sound healing is vast and can be quite intimidating if you don't have some sort of map. Perhaps this book offers that. However, do remember that a map isn't the terrain itself. If you find something out for yourself that goes against anything written here, believe yourself and *your* responses. That's the only truth I know.

As I wrote in the beginning of this book, despite all the information about sound that I possess, if I don't experience it, then it isn't true for me. That goes for you as well. Honor who you are and what you are . . . and in particular, honor whatever experiences you may have with *the sound.* It's the greatest teacher there is.

Enjoy your continued exploration of the magnificent world of sound. Use these secrets and have a good time!

About the CD *Peaceful Journey*

As the composer of more than 20 recordings, I felt that it was important for me to create the most effective sounds to accompany *The 7 Secrets of Sound Healing.* I wanted to create something new and yet time tested.

The accompanying CD features elements that provide an excellent example of what I consider to be the best use of the information in these pages. Sometimes I feel like a scientist in a sound laboratory, mixing and matching different mantras, tones, and frequencies together. As I mentioned, more than 20 different recordings of mine have been released, but I probably have another 100 completed that haven't been released because they didn't meet my standards.

First and foremost, I always use myself to test the effectiveness of a recording. Then I involve my wife, Andi. After we're both satisfied with it, we then have others experience the music and give us feedback. If the recording meets all of these prerequisites, receiving positive feedback from all who listen to it, it's then released.

I'm very happy to say that I believe this new recording, *Peaceful Journey*—created especially for this book—is among my favorites. In fact, I've been so pleased with it that I've engaged the same methodology to create an entire CD that will be released on its own. The recording of *Peaceful Journey* included herein is designed as a gentle yet powerful tool for enhancing relaxation, combining both the art and science of sound healing to produce a profoundly soothing effect for listeners.

Peaceful Journey uses gentle ambient music that pulses very slowly to decrease your heart rate and breathing patterns. In addition, it employs specific psychoacoustic tones and frequencies that will help entrain your brain waves and synchronize your nervous system with the calm and relaxing sounds on it.

This CD is useful for many purposes, including:

- Inducing calmness and relaxation

- Reducing stress

- Enhancing sleep

- Slowing your heart rate, breathing, and brain-wave activity

- Balancing the hemispheres of the brain

As you listen to this recording, you'll first hear the sound of running water, which assists in slowing down your brain waves to theta/delta range using the phenomenon described in the sonic-entrainment section of Chapter 5. After that, you'll hear the sounds of Tibetan bowls—a sacred and ancient sonic tool with the extraordinary ability to enhance relaxation—which are used through this recording. Next, you'll hear gentle instrumental music utilizing the sounds of flute, zither, harp, and other instruments. Underneath this is the very subtle sound of many voices intoning the sacred mantra *Om* in the 2:3 ratio.

There are also silent affirmations that you won't be able to hear, but which will help encode this recording with the energy of positive intent, affecting your subconscious in a positive and beneficial manner. These affirmations are:

- I am calm and relaxed.

- I feel peace and inner harmony.

- My body is relaxed and at ease.

- My mind is calm and peaceful.

- My heart is open and loving.

- Every day, in every way, I am getting better and better.

- I am healthy, happy, and delighted to be alive.

For optimum results, when first listening to *Peaceful Journey,* it's recommended that you find a comfortable place where you won't be disturbed. This CD is designed to help calm and relax you, so allow yourself the time to fully experience it. Make a commitment to yourself that you won't answer the phone or do any other activity that could possibly distract you from receiving the soothing effects of this recording. You may find that the use of headphones enhances your experience.

Peaceful Journey may also be used as gentle background music in your home or workplace (if this is appropriate for you—please heed the closing note stating that this recording isn't suitable for use while driving or at other times when your focus is needed).

These are suggestions that may help enhance the effects of *Peaceful Journey;* however, it's not necessary to do anything at all when listening to it except enjoy the tones and the experience. By their very nature, the sounds on this recording will help enhance calmness and tranquility within you.

Joining me on this CD are musicians who are all masterful sound healers, including Sarah Benson, Laraaji, and Andi

Goldman. Before we began recording, we all meditated and prayed to be the highest conduits of healing energy. I hope that we have succeeded.

All of the sounds on *Peaceful Journey* work together, employing the 7 Secrets found in this book. The powerful and sacred psychoacoustic tools are useful to create a synergistic effect that's wonderful for both healing and transformation. I trust that you'll enjoy the soothing tranquility of these sounds.

Note: Listening to this recording is excellent for deep relaxation, stress reduction, and meditation. Please do not listen to this CD while driving or operating heavy machinery.

· ● **●** ● ● ·

Recommended Resources

Suggested Reading

Healing Sounds, by Jonathan Goldman (Inner Traditions, 2002)

Shifting Frequencies, by Jonathan Goldman (Light Technology, 1998)

Tantra of Sound, by Jonathan Goldman and Andi Goldman (Hampton Roads, 2005)

Music and Sound in the Healing Arts, by John Beaulieu (Station Hill, 1995)

Sounds of Healing, by Mitchell L. Gaynor, M.D. (Broadway, 1999)

The Healing Forces of Music, by Randall McClellan, Ph.D. (iUniverse, 2000)

Sacred Sounds, by Ted Andrews (Llewellyn, 2001)

Music: Physician for Times to Come, edited by Don Campbell (Quest Books, 1991)

The Power of Sound, by Joshua Leeds (Inner Traditions, 2001)

Toning: The Creative Power of the Voice, by Laurel Elizabeth Keyes (DeVorss, 1973)

Healing with the Voice, by James D'Angelo (HarperCollins, 2001)

The Mozart Effect, by Don Campbell (Avon Books, 1997)

Suggested Listening

Recordings by Jonathan Goldman
Chakra Chants (vol. 1 and 2)
The Lost Chord
Reiki Chants
Medicine Buddha

Ultimate Om
Holy Harmony
The Divine Name (with Gregg Braden)
Tantra of Sound Harmonizer (with Andi Goldman)
Sacred Gateways
Dolphins Dreams
Celestial Yoga
The Angel and the Goddess
Frequencies
ChakraDance
De-Stress
Waves of Light
Celestial Reiki (vol. 1 and 2; with Laraaji and Sarah Benson)

Recordings by Others

Angels of the Deep, by Raphael
Chakra Suite, by Steven Halpern
Tao of Healing, by Dean Evenson, with Li Xiangting
Music for the Mozart Effect, vol. II: Heal the Body, by Don Campbell
Flutes of Interior Time, by Sarah Benson
Self-Healing with Sound & Music, by Andrew Weil, M.D., and Kimba Arem
Ambient 1: Music for Airports, by Brian Eno
Dai Ko Myo, by Weave
Rain of Blessings, by Lama Gyurme and Jean-Philippe Rykiel
Ancient, by Kitaro
Hearing Solar Winds, by David Hykes and the Harmonic Choir
Tibetan Master Chants, by Lama Tashi
Sacred Tibet, by the Gyume Monks
Tibetan Tantric Choir, by the Gyuto Monks
Cascade, by Laraaji
Ambient Support for Learning, Working, and Creating, by Tom Kenyon
Isle of Skye, by Jeffrey Thompson

• ● •

For more information about Jonathan Goldman's books, CDs, and other sonic tools for transformation, as well as additional information on the therapeutic and transformational uses of sound and music, please contact:

Healing Sounds
(800) 246-9764
www.healingsounds.com
info@healingsounds.com

For information on the Sound Healers Association, including material on finding and networking with sound healers, as well as many other resources, please contact:

Sound Healers Association
(303) 443-8181
www.soundhealersassociation.org

• • ● ● • •

Acknowledgments

The list of people I'd like to thank would extend far beyond the covers of this book, for there have been so many whose help I am grateful for, not only with this project, but with all the assorted projects that have manifested throughout the years, and continue to manifest.

My deepest thanks go to my beloved wife, Andi, whose companionship, compassion, kindness, and wisdom have guided me throughout this book and my life with her. In addition, acknowledgments go out to my son, Joshua, and all my family. Thanks to Sarah Benson, Andi Goldman, and Laraaji for their contributions to *Peaceful Journey*. Finally, thanks to Kimba Arem, Gregg Braden, Vickie Dodd, Charles Eagle, Alex Freemon, Dr. John Galm, Jill Kramer, Charles McStravick, Deb and Ed Shapiro, Alec Sims, and the Hay House family—and all the beings who manifest Light & Love through Sound for the fruition of this project.

· · ● ● ● · ·

About the Author

Jonathan Goldman is considered to be one of the founders of modern sound healing, pioneering the field for more than 25 years. An award-winning musician and writer, he's the author of four books and more than 20 CDs. His work combines the spiritual and scientific aspects of sound as a healing and transformational modality.

A former blues and rock musician and filmmaker, Jonathan had a transformational experience that changed his life. In the 1980s, he founded both the Sound Healers Association, which he directs, dedicated to education about and awareness of sound and music for healing, and Spirit Music, of which he is CEO, producing music for meditation, relaxation, and self-transformation. Jonathan received a master's degree from Lesley University, researching the uses of sound and music for healing. He has worked with masters of sound from both the scientific and spiritual traditions and has been empowered by the Dalai Lama's chant master of the Drepung Loseling Monastery to teach Tibetan overtone chanting. He also is a lecturing member of the International Society for Music and Medicine.

A writer, musician, and teacher, Jonathan has written several books, including *Healing Sounds, Shifting Frequencies,* and *Tantra of Sound* (co-authored with his wife, Andi), which won the Visionary Award for "Best Alternative Health Book." His cutting-edge, award-winning recordings include *Chakra Chants, The Lost Chord, The Divine Name* (with Gregg Braden), *Frequencies,* and *Reiki Chants.* His *Ultimate Om* CD was named one of the Top 20 New Age CDs. In addition, his CD collaboration with Tibetan chant master Lama Tashi, *Tibetan Master Chants,* was nominated for a 2006 Grammy Award for "Best Traditional World Music."

An internationally acknowledged master teacher, Jonathan facilitates Healing Sounds Seminars at universities, hospitals, holistic-health centers, and expos throughout the United States and Europe. He has appeared on national television and radio, including Art Bell's *Coast to Coast AM,* and has been featured in periodicals, including *USA Today* and *The New York Times.* His annual Healing Sounds Intensive program attracts participants from throughout the world.

For further information, please contact Jonathan's office:

Healing Sounds
P.O. Box 2240
Boulder, CO 80306
(800) 246-9764 or (303) 443-8181 (international)
E-mail: info@healingsounds.com
Website: **www.healingsounds.com**

Notes

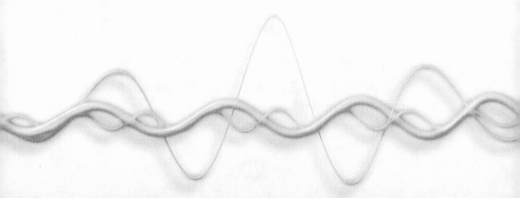

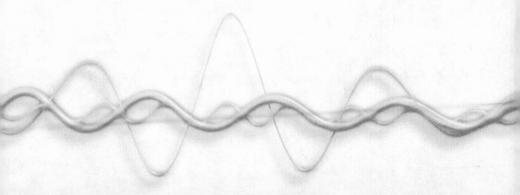

Hay House Titles of Related Interest

YOU CAN HEAL YOUR LIFE, the movie, starring Louise L. Hay & Friends
(available as a 1-DVD program and an expanded 2-DVD set)
Watch the trailer at: **www.LouiseHayMovie.com**

THE SHIFT, the movie,
starring Dr. Wayne W. Dyer
(available as a 1-DVD program and an expanded 2-DVD set)
Watch the trailer at: **www.DyerMovie.com**

• ● •

*CREATING INNER HARMONY: Using Your Voice and Music
to Heal,* by Don Campbell (book-with-CD)

*FOLLOWING SOUND INTO SILENCE: Chanting Your Way Beyond Ego
into Bliss,* by Kurt (Kailash) A. Bruder (book-with-CD)

*LOVE YOUR VOICE: Use Your Speaking Voice to Create Success,
Self-Confidence, and Star-like Charisma!,* by Roger Love
(book-with-CD)

*THE POWER OF INFINITE LOVE & GRATITUDE: An Evolutionary Journey
to Awakening Your Spirit,* by Dr. Darren R. Weissman

RICHES WITHIN: Your Seven Secret Treasures,
by Dr. John F. Demartini

*THE SPONTANEOUS HEALING OF BELIEF: Shattering the Paradigm
of False Limits,* by Gregg Braden

All of the above are available at your local bookstore,
or may be ordered by contacting Hay House (see next page).

• • •

We hope you enjoyed this Hay House book.
If you'd like to receive our online catalog featuring additional information on
Hay House books and products, or if you'd like to find out more about the
Hay Foundation, please contact:

Hay House, Inc.
P.O. Box 5100
Carlsbad, CA 92018-5100

(760) 431-7695 or **(800) 654-5126**
(760) 431-6948 (fax) or **(800) 650-5115 (fax)**
www.hayhouse.com® • **www.hayfoundation.org**

• • •

Published and distributed in Australia by: Hay House Australia Pty. Ltd.,
18/36 Ralph St., Alexandria NSW 2015 • *Phone:* 612-9669-4299 • *Fax:* 612-9669-4144 •
www.hayhouse.com.au

Published and distributed in the United Kingdom by: Hay House UK, Ltd., 292B
Kensal Rd., London W10 5BE • *Phone:* 44-20-8962-1230 • *Fax:* 44-20-8962-1239 •
www.hayhouse.co.uk

Published and distributed in the Republic of South Africa by: Hay House SA (Pty), Ltd.,
P.O. Box 990, Witkoppen 2068 • *Phone/Fax:* 27-11-467-8904 • info@hayhouse.co.za •
www.hayhouse.co.za

Published in India by: Hay House Publishers India, Muskaan Complex, Plot No. 3,
B-2, Vasant Kunj, New Delhi 110 070 • *Phone:* 91-11-4176-1620 • *Fax:* 91-11-4176-1630 •
www.hayhouse.co.in

Distributed in Canada by: Raincoast, 9050 Shaughnessy St., Vancouver, B.C. V6P 6E5 •
Phone: (604) 323-7100 • *Fax:* (604) 323-2600 • www.raincoast.com

• • •

Take Your Soul on a Vacation

Visit **www.HealYourLife.com®** to regroup, recharge, and reconnect with
your own magnificence. Featuring blogs, mind-body-spirit news,
and life-changing wisdom from Louise Hay and friends.

Visit **www.HealYourLife.com today!**

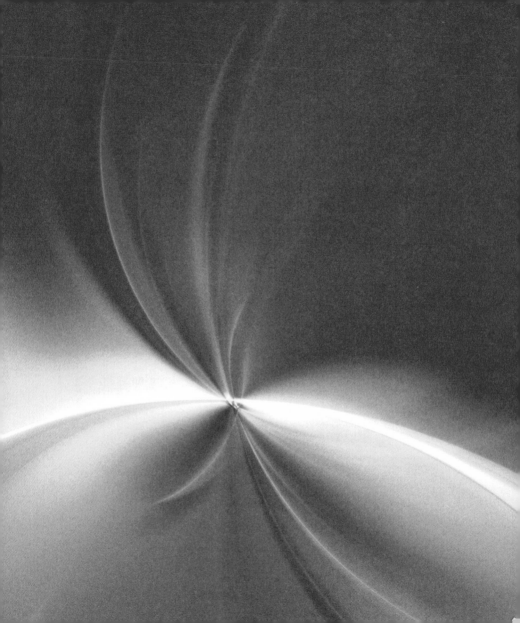